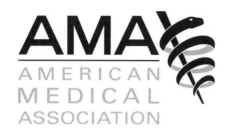

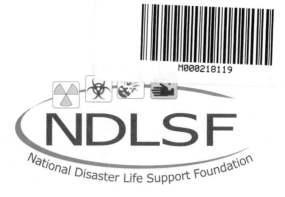

CORE DISASTER LIFE SUPPORT®

v.3.0

Course Manual

Co-Editors-in-Chief

Phillip L. Coule, MD

John A. Mitas II, MD

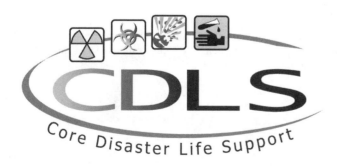

American Medical Association
Executive Vice President, Chief Executive Officer: James L. Madara, MD
Chief Operating Officer: Bernard L. Hengesbaugh
Senior Vice President, Publishing and Business Services: Robert A. Musacchio, PhD
Senior Vice President, Professional Standards: Modena H. Wilson, MD, MPH
Vice President, Science, Medicine and Public Health: Saul Levin, MD, MPA
Director, Center for Public Health Preparedness and Disaster Response:
    James J. James, MD, DrPH, MHA
Vice President, Publications and Clinical Solutions: Mary Lou White
Vice President, Business Operations: Vanessa Hayden
Managing Editor: Janet Thron
Manager, Book and Product Development and Production: Nancy Baker
Director, Sales, Marketing and Strategic Relationships: Joann Skiba
Senior Developmental Editor: Michael Ryder
Production Specialist: Sharon Potter
Marketing Manager: Lori Hollacher

The authors, editors, and publisher of this work have checked with sources believed to be reliable in their efforts to confirm the accuracy and completeness of the information presented herein and that the information is in accordance with the standard practices accepted at the time of publication. However, neither the authors nor the publisher nor any party involved in the creation and publication of this work warrant that the information is in every respect accurate and complete, and they are not responsible for any errors or omissions or for any consequences from application of the information in this book.

Core Disaster Life Support v.3.0

CDLS®, Core Disaster Life Support®, and PRE-DISASTER Paradigm™ are trademarks of the American Medical Association.

ADLS®, BDLS®, DISASTER Paradigm™, Advanced Disaster Life Support™, Basic Disaster Life Support™, National Disaster Life Support™, and NDLSF™ are trademarks of the National Disaster Life Support Foundation, Inc.

Internet address: www.ama-assn.org

BP09:09-P-039.03/10:09
ISBN 978-1-60359-208-6
OP426710

TABLE OF CONTENTS

CHAPTER | ONE

Overview of Disasters and Public Health Emergencies

CHAPTER | **TWO**
Personal Preparedness

CHAPTER | **THREE**
Community Preparation and Planning

CHAPTER | **FOUR**

The Disaster Health System

CHAPTER | **FIVE**

Public Health Law and Ethics

CHAPTER | **SIX**

The DISASTER Paradigm™

Glossary

Appendices:

Index

PREFACE

Disasters affect hundreds of thousands of people every year across the globe. The importance of training to respond appropriately to such events cannot be overemphasized. The National Disaster Life Support Program, a joint effort of the National Disaster Life Support Foundation, Inc., and the American Medical Association, is dedicated to providing educational programs to assist responders and health providers to render the best care possible amidst the chaos that is the disaster.

This course manual is intended as a reference and resource, and therefore it contains more information than can be included in the Core Disaster Life Support® (CDLS®) course. This information will be valuable to disaster-response professionals in their preparedness planning.

The CDLS course is a competency-based, awareness-level course aimed at a broad range of audiences, including medical first responders, health professionals, health service providers, public health workers, and health support personnel. It provides the common vocabulary and working knowledge necessary to help ensure that all potential health system responders understand their role and how it is integrated with other segments of the disaster response system. The CDLS course teaches the "all-hazards" approach to personal, institutional, and community disaster management through the introduction of two unique mnemonics:

> ➤ The PRE-DISASTER Paradigm™ (which applies to event mitigation and preparedness); and

> ➤ The DISASTER Paradigm™ (which applies to event recognition, response, and recovery).

The CDLS course lays the foundation for individuals from diverse professions, disciplines, and backgrounds to come together as a team to enhance personal and community preparedness and resilience for catastrophic health emergencies. It provides a framework to enable public health, emergency medical services, and other response personnel to work as partners in local preparedness and response efforts.

The editors and contributors trust that you will find this manual a valuable resource, both for the CDLS course and as a reference.

Phillip L. Coule, MD,
Co-Editor-in-Chief, Core Disaster Life Support®

John A. Mitas, II, MD
Co-Editor-in-Chief, Core Disaster Life Support®

ACKNOWLEDGMENTS

CONTRIBUTING EDITORS

Italo Subbarao, DO, MBA
Jim Lyznicki, MS, MPH

The American Medical Association and the National Disaster Life Support Foundation, Inc., extend sincere appreciation to the founding authors and editors of the National Disaster Life Support™ course curricula for their continued vision and leadership in advancing and promoting excellence in education and training of all health professionals in disaster medicine and public health preparedness:

Phillip L. Coule, MD
Cham E. Dallas, PhD
James J. James, MD, DrPH, MHA
Scott Lillibridge, MD
Paul E. Pepe, MD, MPH
Richard B. Schwartz, MD
Raymond E. Swienton, MD

Developed in collaboration with:

The National Disaster Life Support Education Consortium™
Medical College of Georgia
University of Texas, Southwestern Medical Center at Dallas
University of Texas, School of Public Health at Houston
University of Georgia

Special Acknowledgment

The Co-Editors and the American Medical Association (AMA) Center for Public Health Preparedness and Disaster Response wish to acknowledge the special contribution of Jessica Sempek, MS, Program Administrator, AMA National Disaster Life Support Program Office.

In addition, we thank the National Disaster Life Support Education Consortium for their support of this project.

ABOUT THE CO-EDITORS-IN-CHIEF

Phillip L. Coule, MD, is one of the original creators of the National Disaster Life Support™ (NDLS™) series of courses and with colleagues developed the concept of the DISASTER Paradigm™. Dr. Coule, a former emergency medical technician (EMT), remains involved in pre-hospital emergency and disaster care. He is the former director of the Center of Operational Medicine at the Georgia Health Sciences University and currently serves as the vice-chairman for Business Development and Professor of Emergency Medicine.

John A. Mitas II, MD, is special advisor to the executive vice president of the American College of Physicians after serving as chief operating officer and deputy executive vice president from 2002 to 2009. He is board certified in Internal Medicine and Nephrology and retired from the Navy after 30 years in academic, senior executive, and operational medicine positions, including humanitarian relief missions and Commanding Officer of the hospital in USNS COMFORT.

ABOUT THE CONTRIBUTING EDITORS AND CONTRIBUTORS

Contributing Editors:

Italo Subbarao, DO, MBA, is the director of the Public Health Readiness Office at the AMA Center for Public Health Preparedness and Disaster Response, the deputy editor of *Disaster Medicine and Public Health Preparedness*, and the medical director, National Disaster Life Support Program Office. Dr. Subbarao has expertise in health system recovery and promoting comprehensive disaster planning through private-public partnerships.

Jim Lyznicki, MS, MPH, is the associate director of the Center for Public Health Preparedness and Disaster Response at the American Medical Association. He holds master's degrees in medical microbiology and in environmental and occupational health.

Contributors:

Frederick M. Burkle, Jr., MD, MPH, DTM, is senior fellow, the Harvard Humanitarian Initiative, Harvard School of Public Health and senior associate faculty and research scientist, the Center for Refugee and Disaster Response, Johns Hopkins University Medical Institutes. He also serves as a senior public policy scholar, Woodrow Wilson Center for International Scholars, Washington, DC (2008–2010).

Michael Cronin, PhD, MPH, is a longtime leader in community health, having founded, led, and directed a cutting-edge nonprofit health and human services agency in Boston for more than two decades. Today, he holds the position of program manager for the American Trauma Society (ATS), where he serves as ATS's principal investigator for the CDC TIIDE (Terrorist Injuries: Information, Dissemination, and Exchange) Project, as well as serving as senior editor of the International Trauma and Disaster Institute at Massachusetts General Hospital in Boston.

Andrea Garcia, JD, is the director of state government affairs for the American Osteopathic Association. Prior to joining the AOA, Ms. Garcia served as a policy analyst at the American Medical Association (2004–2009), a senior researcher with The Centers for Law and the Public's Health: A Collaborative at Georgetown and Johns Hopkins Universities, and a fellow with the International Weapons Control Center at DePaul University.

E. Brooke Lerner, PhD, is an injury epidemiologist and a former emergency medical services (EMS) field provider. She is currently an associate professor at the Medical College of Wisconsin in the Department of Emergency Medicine. She has nearly 20 years of EMS-related experience and has written dozens of EMS-related, peer-reviewed publications.

Jim Lyznicki, MS, MPH, is the associate director of the Center for Public Health Preparedness and Disaster Response at the American Medical Association. He holds master's degrees in medical microbiology and in environmental and occupational health.

David Markenson, MD, is the vice president and medical director for disaster medicine and regional emergency service at Westchester Medical Center and the Maria Fareri Children's Hospital. He also serves as the interim chair and director of the Center for Disaster Medicine at the School of Health Sciences and Practice New York Medical College. Dr. Markenson is a professor of pediatrics and associate professor of public health at New York Medical College.

John F. Ryan, CEM, has spent 26 years with the Department of Defense. He has traveled extensively in support of the NDLSF™ and its programs, both domestically and internationally. John currently serves as chief of special operations for the Fort Gordon Fire and Emergency Services at Fort Gordon near Augusta, GA.

Leslie Gunning-Scofield, BA, NREMT-B, is director for first responder education and Regional Training Center coordinator for National Disaster Life Support™ (NDLS™) programs at the Center for Biopreparedness Education, a joint endeavor between Creighton University Medical Center and the University of Nebraska Medical Center. As director for first responder education, her responsibility involves identifying gaps in knowledge and training needs in the area of disaster preparedeness. Leslie has several years of experience in EMS and adult education.

Greene Shepherd, PharmD, is a professor of clinical pharmacy at the University of Georgia. Dr. Shepherd specializes in clinical toxicology and emergency pharmacy.

Italo Subbarao, DO, MBA, is the director of the Public Health Readiness Office at the AMA Center for Public Health Preparedness and Disaster Response, the deputy editor of *Disaster Medicine and Public Health Preparedness*, and the medical director, National Disaster Life Support Program Office. Dr. Subbarao has expertise in health system recovery and promoting comprehensive disaster planning through private-public partnerships.

REVIEWERS

John H. Armstrong, MD
University of Florida-Gainesville

Mona R. Bomgaars, MD, MPH
American Academy of Family Physicians

Apryl Brown, MD, MPH
Detroit Medical Reserve Corps

Allen Cherson, DO
Medisys Regional NDLS™ Training Center

Arthur Cooper, MD, MS
Columbia University

Kevin Frey, CST, MA
Association of Surgical Technologists

Timothy Gough, RN, BSN, MSN
Ripon Medical Center

J. Brian Houston, PhD
University of Oklahoma Health Sciences Center

Connie Kraft, RN, MSN, CEN
Stony Brook University Medical Center

Ajoy Kumar, MD
Bayfront Family Medicine Residency

Raj Lal, MD, MS, MBA, MPA
Illinois Medical Emergency Response Team

Mary-Elise Manuell, MD, MA
UMass Memorial Medical Center

Edward McGinley, NREMT-P
Tarrant County (TX) Medical Reserve Corps

Jennifer E. Miller, MS
Bioethics International

David Nitsch, BS, NREMT-P
Albert Einstein Medical Center

Kevin O'Hara, MS, EMT-P
Nassau County EMS Academy

Al Osbahr, MD
Catawba Valley Medical Center

David Persaud, BS, RN, EMT-B CHEP
Illinois I Region Hospital Coordination Center

Kevin Reilly, PE, PP, MS, MD
Ireland Army Community Hospital

Jeff Rubin, PhD, CEM
Tualatin Valley Fire and Rescue

Heather Seemann, NREMT-P, FP-C, MLT (ACSP)
Pulaski County Ambulance District

Jonathan Simmons, DO, MS
University of Iowa Hospitals and Clinics

John Snider, RN, CEN, CEM, AEMT
Henry Ford Hospital

Andrew E. Spain, MA, NCEE, EMT-P
University of Missouri

Sharon A. R. Stanley, PhD, RN
American Red Cross

Richard Thomas, PharmD
Primary Children's Medical Center

COURSE OBJECTIVES

Upon completion of the Core Disaster Life Support® (CDLS®) course, participants will be able to:

➤ Describe the all-hazards approach to disaster mitigation, preparedness, response, and recovery.

➤ Discuss essential components of federal, state, regional, and community disaster health systems, including the role of the public and private health sectors.

➤ Describe the elements of the PRE-DISASTER Paradigm™ and their application to the management of disasters and public health emergencies.

➤ Describe actions that can be taken to enhance personal preparedness and resilience for disasters and public health emergencies.

➤ Identify legal and ethical issues that impact disaster mitigation, preparedness, response, and recovery, including the basic legal framework for public health.

➤ Describe the elements of the DISASTER Paradigm™ and their application for the management of disasters and public health emergencies.

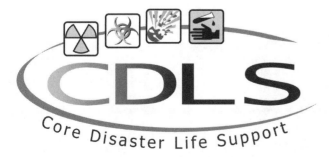

CHAPTER ONE

Overview of Disasters and Public Health Emergencies

1.1 PURPOSE

This chapter provides the definitions, descriptions, and categorization of disasters and public health emergencies for the National Disaster Life Support™ (NDLS™) Program. It also provides an overview of the scope, magnitude, and health implications of these events.

1.2 LEARNING OBJECTIVES

After completing this chapter, readers should be able to:

➤ Given a list of disaster-related terms, match each to its correct definition.

➤ Given a list of disaster events, explain whether the event is most likely a natural or a human-caused event.

➤ Given the PRE-DISASTER Paradigm™, identify each element of the paradigm in the context of the all-hazards framework for disaster management.

➤ Given the DISASTER Paradigm™, identify each element of the paradigm in the context of the all-hazards framework for disaster management.

1.3 DISASTER MEDICINE AND PUBLIC HEALTH PREPAREDNESS COMPETENCY ADDRESSED

This chapter addresses the following competency as delineated in Appendix E of this manual.

➤ Describe the all-hazards framework for disaster planning and mitigation.

1.4 INTRODUCTION

The magnitude and toll of natural disasters and terrorism have increased throughout the world. According to the Center for Research on the Epidemiology of Disasters, in the previous century, about 3.5 million people were killed worldwide as a result of natural disasters; about 200 million were killed as a result of human-caused disasters (eg, war, terrorism, genocide). Each year in the United States, disasters cause hundreds of deaths and cost billions of dollars due to disruption of commerce and destruction of homes and critical infrastructure. Although the number of lives lost to disasters each year generally has declined, the economic cost of major disaster response and recovery continues to rise. Each decade, property damage from these events doubles or triples.

The growing likelihood of terrorist-related disasters affecting large civilian populations has been described in many venues, from professional journals to Congressional hearings to media documentaries. Concern continues about the security of the worldwide arsenal of nuclear, chemical, and biologic agents, as well as the recruitment of people capable of manufacturing or deploying them. While the likelihood of a successful terrorist attack may seem remote compared to other known health risks, the potentially catastrophic nature of such an event demands that health care professionals and their communities be prepared. Natural disasters such as tornadoes, hurricanes, floods, and earthquakes, as well as industrial and transportation-related catastrophes, are far more common and can severely stress existing medical, public health, and emergency response systems. The emergence of infectious diseases, such as novel H1N1 influenza A and severe acute respiratory syndrome (SARS), and the recent arrival of West Nile virus and monkey pox in the Western hemisphere, reinforces the need for constant vigilance and planning to prepare for and respond to new and unexpected public health emergencies.

In light of recent world events, it is increasingly clear that all health professionals need to become more proficient in the recognition, diagnosis, and treatment of mass casualties under an all-hazards approach to disaster management and response. They must be able to recognize the general features of public health emergencies, and be knowledgeable about how to report them and where to get more information should the need arise. Health professionals are on the front lines when dealing with injury and disease—whether caused by microbes, environmental hazards, natural disasters, highway collisions, terrorism, or other calamities. Early detection and reporting are critical to minimize casualties through astute teamwork by public- and private-sector health and emergency response personnel.

1.5 DEFINITIONS AND TERMINOLOGY

Consensus definitions and terminology are extremely important in disaster research for identifying events and data to include or exclude from analysis. If events and data are identified with a common definition, they can be more easily studied and compared; however, many definitions of a disaster exist. The World Association of Disaster and Emergency Medicine (WADEM) defines a *disaster* as a serious disruption of the functioning of society, causing widespread human, material, or environmental losses that exceed the ability of affected society to cope by using only its own resources. A disaster is the result of a vast ecological breakdown in the relations between humans and their environment, a serious and sudden (or slow, as in drought) event on such a scale that the stricken community needs extraordinary efforts to cope with it, often with outside help or international aid. A disaster results when the absorbing capacity of the affected society is unable to maintain the functionality of an essential element above a threshold. WADEM also defines a *health disaster* as a precipitous or gradual decline in the overall health status of a community for which the community is unable to cope without outside assistance.[1]

The US Federal Emergency Management Agency (FEMA) defines a disaster as "an occurrence of a natural catastrophe, technological accident, or human caused event that has resulted in severe property damage, deaths, and/or multiple injuries."

In accordance with the all-hazards framework for disaster management, the NDLS Program promotes the following definition: "An event and its consequences that result in a serious disruption of the functioning of a community and cause widespread human, material, economic, or environmental losses that exceed the capacity of the affected area to respond without external assistance to save lives, preserve property, and maintain the stability and integrity of the affected area." For operational purposes, a disaster can be defined as "an event in which the needs exceed immediately available resources."

1.5.1 Time-Limited Disasters

A time-limited disaster is generally defined as being less than 72 hours in duration. A typical example is a tornado, bombing, or explosion. Such events may be referred to as mass casualty incidents (MCIs) or mass casualty events (MCEs), since they may involve multiple direct traumatic injuries and deaths. Some organizations, such as the American College of Surgeons, make a distinction between MCIs and MCEs on the basis of casualty flow and strain on the local and regional health care systems. In this classification an MCI is defined as 5 or more patients from an incident that strains the local health care system. An MCE is defined as an event involving 20 or more patients that overwhelms the regional health system. Though local health care and emergency response systems may be overwhelmed for a few hours, the public health infrastructure usually remains intact and the system stabilizes approximately 4 to 6 hours after the event.

1.5.2   Prolonged Disasters and Public Health Emergencies

A large-scale or prolonged disaster may warrant being termed a public health emergency if it significantly destroys and/or disrupts (1) the public health infrastructure and system (which includes both private and public hospitals and health care systems, emergency medical services systems, and local public health agencies); and (2) the protections the public health infrastructure and system provide to a population. These protections, traditionally known as *essential public health services*, provide for clean water, sanitation, food, health services, shelter, and fuel (essential to avoid temperature extremes). Also included are essential public health system services such as disease surveillance and access and availability to health services. Some of these protections are lost if populations are forced to flee, when populations either are internally displaced within their own country or cross international borders as refugees.

Whereas a disaster event itself results in *direct* deaths, injuries, or illnesses, public health emergencies are measured by the *indirect* consequences they cause. These indirect deaths (mortality) and illnesses (morbidity) are often referred to as *excess mortality and morbidity* and would have been preventable had the need for public health measures been predicted or managed. Indirect consequences often define gaps in disaster preparedness and response systems. For example, in 2005, Hurricane Katrina resulted in approximately 1500 direct deaths due to the storm and flooding; however, indirect deaths may have exceeded direct deaths. An analysis of obituaries reported to the local newspaper suggests a dramatic rise in death rates in New Orleans following Hurricane Katrina, most likely due to a lack of access to and availability of numerous public health protections.[2] Even the health surveillance system was destroyed and failed to identify, monitor, and evaluate causes of actual and potential mortality and morbidity that occurred for months after the disaster event itself. The indirect consequences resulting from a destroyed, compromised, poorly maintained, or poorly repaired public health infrastructure and system may be seen in large-scale natural disasters, war, political violence and conflict, and epidemics and pandemics, as well as in unintentional or intentional biologic, chemical, and radiation or nuclear events.

Public health emergencies require a dramatic shift in health-related decision making from conventional individual- or patient-centered approaches to decisions that consider the well-being of entire communities and populations (called *population-based care*). To minimize indirect consequences such as excess deaths and morbidity, scarce resources may be provided only to persons who have the best opportunity for survival. Communities may have to ration resources and increase capacity to accommodate the increased patient volume. The ability of a health care system to increase capacity to care for large numbers of patients from a disaster is referred to as *surge capacity*. The prioritization of care for patients based on the severity of their illness or injury, their ability to survive, and the resources available is referred to as *triage*.

In a public health emergency, limitations in clinical and public health resources may involve difficult moral and ethical decisions. Citizen understanding and acceptance of these decisions is critical and requires that local health authorities and emergency planners consider the needs and concerns of members of both genders, all ages, and vulnerable populations in advance of any serious emergency. In 2003, the Toronto experience with the SARS outbreak affirmed that citizens can comprehend the need for health rationing in a serious emergency. In a large-scale disease outbreak, few, if any, local public health systems and infrastructures have the requisite resources to deal with all health-related demands. Recent examples of disasters that have become public health emergencies include the Indonesian tsunami (2004), Hurricanes Katrina and Rita (2005), the Pakistan earthquake (2008), Hurricane Ike (2008), Cyclone Nargis (2008), the Sichuan earthquake (2008), and the novel H1N1 influenza A pandemic (2009), and the Haitian earthquake (2010).

1.6 DISASTER TYPOLOGY

A number of disaster classifications exist. The most inclusive taxonomy defines three distinct categories (natural disasters, human systems [technological] failure, and war and conflict) as one dimension of classification and time as another dimension (time-limited vs prolonged disasters). Disasters can overlap categories. For example, Hurricane Katrina was a natural disaster, but the levee breaches and delayed response could be considered human systems failures. Generally, a disaster is classified according to its primary categorization, and so Hurricane Katrina would be considered a natural disaster.

It is important to recognize the important distinction between hazards and disasters. Hazards present the possibility for a disaster occurrence caused by natural phenomena or human activities. Whether or not a given hazard causes a disaster will depend on the setting, vulnerability, mitigation, and the resources available to respond to the event. For example, the collapse of a high-rise office building after collision by a jet aircraft carrying 200 passengers would be a disaster for even the most well-prepared, well-equipped, and well-staffed health care system. On the other hand, a single-vehicle collision of a bus on a remote stretch of rural interstate highway, with five fatalities and six surviving victims, would likely represent a disaster for most small community hospitals without trauma services capacity. For a large metropolitan area, a similar event would likely be handled as a matter of routine response.

1.6.1   All-Hazards Preparedness

All-hazards preparedness refers to considering all potential hazards to a community and taking steps to mitigate, prepare, and respond to any potential hazard that may affect the community. Single-hazard–focused preparedness is dependent on correct anticipation of the next disaster that may impact the community. This approach can leave significant gaps in preparedness. By considering and preparing the community for all hazards, gaps in response plans can be lessened, potentially resulting in a better response to the event.

Disaster Category	Examples
Natural	➤ Earthquake ➤ Hurricane ➤ Landslide ➤ Tornado ➤ Volcano ➤ Natural outbreak of infectious disease
Human systems failure	➤ Airplane crash ➤ Chemical release/spill ➤ Nuclear plant meltdown ➤ Train derailment ➤ Building collapse
Conflict	➤ Civil disturbance ➤ Complex emergency ➤ Terrorism (including bioterrorism) ➤ War

The distinction between natural and technological (human-caused) disasters can become blurred, as in the case of industrial catastrophes, structural collapse of buildings, transportation-related emergencies, release of hazardous materials by fires or explosions, and infectious disease outbreaks. Dealing with these commonly occurring events requires an all-hazards approach to disaster management to better coordinate planning and response assets.

In recent years, use of the expression *natural disasters* has come under some scrutiny, as it conveys the mistaken assumption that disasters occurring as a result of natural hazards are wholly "natural" and therefore inevitable and outside of human control. To a large extent, disasters are determined by human action, or lack thereof. Natural hazards can seriously impact a community or region, leading to economic and ecological disruption and human suffering that cannot be alleviated without extraordinary assistance from outside the affected community or region. The resulting loss depends on the capacity of the affected population to support or resist the disaster, and the population's resilience. The risks and potential for disasters associated with natural hazards are largely shaped by existing levels of vulnerability and measures that are taken to prevent, mitigate, and prepare for these events. The expression *disasters associated with natural hazards* therefore has been proposed as more appropriate terminology, but for simplicity this text will refer to such events as "natural disasters." However, the reader is encouraged to remember that all consequences associated with these events are not directly caused by the event itself and that one should consider the broader term.

1.7 NATURE AND SCOPE OF DISASTERS AND PUBLIC HEALTH EMERGENCIES

According to the World Health Organization (WHO) Center for Research on the Epidemiology of Disasters (WHO CRED), the frequency of disasters worldwide has doubled since 1995. Part of the increase is attributed to better reporting due to improved surveillance and communication technologies such as the Internet and cellular telephones. Global trends indicate that the frequency and magnitude (and thus the risk) of disaster hazards is on the rise. Population vulnerability (eg, due to urbanization and overpopulation) has increased the risk of disasters and public health emergencies. Globalization, which connects countries through economic interdependencies, has led to increased international travel and commerce. Such activity also has led to overpopulation in cities around the world and increased movement of people to coastal areas and other disaster-prone regions. Increases in international travel may speed the rate at which an emerging infectious disease or bioterrorism agent spreads across the globe. Climate change and terrorism have emerged as important global factors that can influence disaster trends and thus require continued monitoring and attention.

Without question, a disaster will occur somewhere in the United States every year. Intensive monitoring by federal agencies such as the Centers for Disease Control and Prevention (CDC), National Weather Service, National Oceanic and Atmospheric Administration, US Department of Homeland Security, and US Geological Survey can provide early warning of some of these events. This facilitates disaster mitigation by allowing implementation of emergency plans

Center for Research on the Epidemiology of Disasters (CRED)

The CRED was established in 1973 as a nonprofit institution located within the School of Public Health of the University Catholique de Louvain in Brussels, Belgium. CRED became a WHO Collaborating Center in 1980 and has expanded its support of the WHO Global Program for Emergency Preparedness and Response. The center focuses on health aspects and impacts from disasters and complex emergencies. These include all types of natural and human-caused events, longer-term disasters such as famines and droughts, and situations creating mass displacement of people such as civil strife and conflicts.

For more information, refer to the CRED Web site at http://www.cred.be/.

and evacuations. Although some disasters are predictable according to season or geographic location and through the use of sophisticated tracking systems, many others can occur with little or no warning.

1.8   NATURAL DISASTERS[3-7]

In 2008, natural disasters occurred in more than 350 countries, caused more than 235,000 deaths, and affected more than 214 million people.[3] Economic damages were projected at $190 billion dollars. Statistics from prior years are shown in Figure 1-1 and Table 1-1.

Most natural disasters are limited in duration and do not become public health emergencies. According to the WHO CRED database, more natural disasters occur in Asia than other continents; China experiences the most natural disasters. The CRED database also shows that the most common type of disaster throughout the United States and the world is floods (Figure 1-2).

After a primary natural disaster, responders must be prepared for subsequent or secondary emergencies. Special attention must be given to structural collapse, downed power lines, ruptured gas lines, and loss of other basic services. While a building may sustain no immediately apparent effects during a disaster, it may still be structurally damaged or otherwise unstable enough to pose a serious risk for its inhabitants, with a need for evacuation. The consequences of prolonged power outages, contaminated drinking water supplies, and infectious disease outbreaks also must be considered. Natural disasters pose a substantial risk of communications disruptions, infrastructure destruction, and large numbers of displaced persons who require food, shelter, and medical care. Moreover, they may create a need for resources not commonly considered in disaster response. For example, building collapse after an earthquake requires rapid mobilization

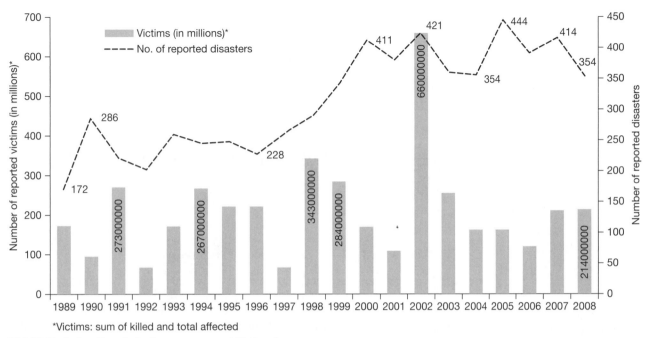

FIGURE 1-1 Trends in Occurrence and Victims[3]

of construction personnel and heavy equipment, urban search and rescue teams, and mortuary services.

1.8.1 Drought and Famine

Drought is a normal, recurrent feature of climate. It occurs almost everywhere, although its features vary from region to region. In the most general sense, drought originates from a deficiency of precipitation over an extended period of time, resulting in water shortages that can have a dire impact on agricultural, environmental, and other resources. Droughts can be complex

TABLE 1-1 Global Natural Disaster Statistics for the 21st Century[3]

Natural Disaster Impact	2008	2000–2007 Average
Number of country-level disasters	354	397
Number of countries affected	133	116.3
Number of people killed	235,000	66,813
Number of people affected	214 million	234 million
Economic damage (US dollars)	$190 billion	$82 billion

FIGURE 1-2

Occurrence of Natural
Disasters by Type and Year[3]

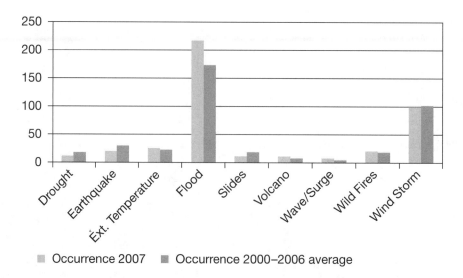

in origin because they often occur as a result of the interplay between a prolonged decrease in precipitation and human demands for food and water in the affected region.

In 2008, more than 13 drought-related disasters were reported worldwide. In the United States, no drought-related fatalities were reported in 2008; however, drought-related damages totaled $1.7 million.

1.8.2   Earthquakes

Earthquakes are among the most devastating natural disasters. Not every earthquake, however, causes a disaster. Numerous imperceptible earthquakes occur almost daily in many regions of the United States. Massive earthquakes, however, cause enormous devastation. Loss of life, property, and infrastructure, as well as the economic impact on affected communities, can be overwhelming.

Earthquakes strike with no warning and can occur at any time of the year and at any time of day or night. The precise geologic cause is still unknown, although a significant factor is the shifting of tectonic plates that form the earth's crust. Stress at fault lines where these plates meet causes them to rupture, releasing enormous quantities of energy as a seismic wave that causes significant shaking and physical damage at the earth's surface. This shaking can cause buildings and bridges to collapse and can create secondary disasters such as flooding, landslides, and tsunamis, which can take a heavy toll on areas already devastated by the original earthquake. Secondary disasters can also include downed power lines, ruptured gas and water lines, explosions, and fires. The point of rupture is known as the focus, and the epicenter is the area on the surface directly above the underground focus. Despite constant monitoring of seismic activity and geographic features, the ability to predict or detect a significant earthquake in time to warn communities and to mitigate its effects is limited.

Earthquake intensity is measured by the Richter scale, which ranges from 0 to 10. Earthquakes of magnitude 6 or greater are generally considered significant. Each year, 70 to 75 damaging earthquakes occur throughout the world. Geographically, the Asian Pacific Rim from Japan to Indonesia—part of the Pacific Ring of Fire—is the most seismically active area in the world.

In 2008, there were 23 disasters attributable to earthquakes worldwide. The 2008 Sichuan earthquake in China measured 8.0 on the Richter scale and caused more than 80,000 deaths. The United States is seismically quite active; only a fraction of its fault lines have been identified and mapped. The most recent US earthquake disaster was the 1994 Northridge earthquake in California, which measured 6.8 on the Richter scale (57 fatalities, about 9000 injured). After the earthquake, a total of 24,000 dwellings were vacated. The total cost of the earthquake was estimated to be at least $10 billion, which makes it one of the most expensive natural disasters in US history. Most earthquake-related fatalities are due to direct trauma.

1.8.3   Extreme Heat

Extreme heat is defined as a prolonged period of temperatures that are 10°F or more above the average high temperature for the region. The heat index is a temperature expressed in degrees Fahrenheit that is derived from the combination of relative humidity and air temperature.

US Geological Survey

Part of the US Department of the Interior, the US Geological Survey (USGS) collects, monitors, analyzes, and provides scientific understanding about natural resource conditions, issues, and problems. A major goal of the USGS is to reduce the vulnerability of the people and areas most at risk from natural hazards. The USGS is one of four federal agencies contributing to the National Earthquake Hazards Reduction Program, the other three being FEMA, the National Science Foundation, and the National Institute of Standards and Technology. The USGS Earthquake Hazards program (http://earthquake.usgs.gov/) and Volcano Hazards Program (http://volcanoes .usgs.gov/) provide up-to-date global information about seismic and volcanic activity, respectively. The USGS also provides timely information on wildfires, hurricanes, floods/drought, and tsunamis. For more information about the USGS, refer to the Web site at http://www.usgs.gov/.

The National Weather Service

Housed within the National Oceanic and Atmospheric Administration (NOAA), the National Weather Service provides weather, hydrologic, and climate forecasts and warnings for the United States, its territories, adjacent waters, and ocean areas. The National Weather Service data and products form a national information database and infrastructure that can be used by other governmental agencies, the private sector, the public, and the global community. For additional information, visit the National Weather Service Web site at http://www.nws.noaa.gov/.

Heat is one of the most underrated and least understood of the deadly weather phenomena. In contrast to the visible, destructive, and violent characteristics associated with other natural disasters, such as floods and tornadoes, a heat wave can be a "silent killer." The worst heat disasters, in terms of loss of life, occur in large cities when a combination of high daytime temperatures, high humidity, warm nighttime temperatures, and an abundance of sunshine occurs for several days. Large urban areas become "heat islands." Brick buildings, asphalt streets, and tar roofs store heat and radiate it like a slow-burning furnace. Heat builds up in a city during the day, and cities are slower than rural areas to cool down at night.

According to the National Weather Service, in 2008 there were 217 extreme heat–related injuries and 71 extreme heat–related fatalities in the United States. The 10-year average is 170 fatalities per year, making it the leading weather-related killer. Damages from extreme heat totaled $0.6 million in 2008.

1.8.4   Floods

Flooding is the most common disaster in the world. Ninety percent of all natural disasters in the United States involve flooding. Secondary contamination of water supplies from sewage and vector overgrowth (mosquitoes) from pooling of water are issues of concern. Although floods may be more predictable than some other types of natural disasters, they are largely unpreventable and prolonged. Massive floods evolve rather slowly, often over a period of days, and with some advanced warning, whereas flash floods, as the name implies, develop quickly and involve relatively small volumes of water. Flash floods are a leading weather-related killer in the United States. They can occur within a few minutes or hours of excessive rainfall, a dam or levee failure, or a sudden release of water held by an ice jam. Flash floods are known as "urban rivers." They are slow killers, often with water speeds of no more than 6 to 12 mph. This is deceptive, however; the force generated by only 2 feet of water is sufficient to move an automobile. Flash floods are also known as "blind traps," because underwater debris and road damage increase the potential for injury and death. Many injuries occur when people are walking through flooded areas and are injured by underwater objects.

Each year, an average of 170 people lose their lives in floods, with damage averaging more than $2 billion. The most common flood-related cause of death is drowning, and most injuries result from collision with underwater objects. In 2008, there were more than 166 flooding disasters worldwide. According to FEMA, from January 2000 to March 2007 there were 62 flooding disasters in the United States that required federal assistance. In 2008 there were 82 flood-related deaths in the United States, with 54 attributed to flash flooding.

1.8.5 Tropical Cyclones and Tropical Storms

These are powerful windstorms that develop over warm tropical waters in the southern Atlantic Ocean, Caribbean Sea, and Gulf of Mexico, as well as in the eastern and central Pacific Ocean and Indian Ocean. Tropical cyclones that occur north of the equator and in the Pacific Ocean may be referred to as *typhoons*. For the purposes of this text, *hurricane* should be interpreted to refer to all tropical cyclones, including typhoons. Under the right conditions, tropical cyclones (hurricanes) can produce violent winds, enormous waves, torrential rains, widespread flooding, and tidal surge.

Hurricane intensity and severity are rated from 1 to 5 (according to the Saffir-Simpson scale). Category 3, 4, and 5 storms are considered major hurricanes. In general, the more severe category 5 storms cause more devastation, but even less powerful tropical depressions and tropical storms can be very destructive, largely because of the resultant flooding, landslides, and torrential rain rather than from the high wind speeds and storm surge of more powerful storms (*storm surge* is the onshore rush of water caused by the powerful winds associated with the landfall of a hurricane). These secondary environmental disasters are one of the hallmarks of hurricanes. Hurricanes are typically forecast well in advance, but mitigation and effective response rely on well-coordinated, well-timed evacuations and effective communication.

According to 2008 statistics, there were more than 112 hurricanes/cyclones in the world in that year. The United States experienced 17 tropical storms in the Atlantic Ocean, of which eight became hurricanes (causing 11 deaths). Fatalities in hurricanes generally result from direct traumatic injury and drowning.

The National Hurricane Center

Located within the National Oceanic and Atmospheric Administration, the National Hurricane Center (NHC) seeks to save lives, mitigate property loss, and improve economic efficiency by issuing tropical storm watches, warnings, and forecasts through analysis of hazardous weather patterns, and by increasing understanding of these hazards through global outreach. For additional information, visit the NHC Web site at http://www.nhc.noaa.gov/.

1.8.6   Landslides

Landslides are typically associated with periods of heavy rainfall or rapid snow melt and tend to worsen the effects of flooding that often accompanies these events. In areas burned by forest and brush fires, a lower threshold of precipitation may initiate landslides. Debris flows, sometimes referred to as *mudslides*, mud-flows, lahars (volcanic lava and landslide combined), or *debris avalanches*, are common types of fast-moving landslides. It is estimated that landslides cause up to $2 billion in damages and from 25 to 50 deaths annually in the United States.

1.8.7   Tornadoes

Tornadoes are severe windstorms that are characterized by a rapidly rotating column of air extending from a thunderstorm to the ground. Tornadoes are among the most violent storms. Tornadoes are scaled by wind force on the enhanced Fujita (EF) scale, ranging from 0 to 5. Storms under 85 mph are classified as EF-0; EF-5 refers to tornadoes with winds exceeding 200 mph. The most violent tornadoes are capable of tremendous destruction. Damage paths can be in excess of 1 mile wide and 50 miles long. Tornadoes can occur anywhere in the United States at any time of the year. In the southern states, peak tornado season is March through May, while peak months in the northern states are June, July, and August.

Tornadoes can occur anywhere in the world, but most often they occur in the United States, Europe, and Southeast Asia. The United States has more severe tornadoes than any other country because of climate and terrain. They are most common in the midsection of the country ("tornado alley"). In an average year, about 1000 tornadoes are reported across the United States, resulting in 87 deaths and more than 1500 injuries.

A category EF-5 tornado with winds in excess of 250 mph will destroy mobile homes, level buildings, and hurl automobiles into the air as missiles. In addition to fatalities and injuries, the severe structural damage can present long-term recovery issues for affected communities. Tornadoes also pose a significant risk of secondary disasters due to structural collapses, explosions, and fires.

1.8.8   Tsunamis

The word *tsunami* originates from the Japanese words *tsu*, meaning "harbor," and *nami*, meaning "wave." Tsunamis (commonly but incorrectly called *tidal waves*) are a series of long waves that can travel thousands of miles across the open ocean but become concentrated when they impact shores and can be concentrated in harbors—thus the origin of the name "harbor wave." Most tsunamis are generated by sea floor displacements from large undersea earthquakes, but they can also originate from submarine landslides caused by earthquakes or undersea volcanoes. The waves can travel across the ocean nearly undetectable but release their energy as they impact the shoreline, potentially decimating entire villages and sweeping victims out to sea.

Tsunamis can cause considerable destruction and loss of life within minutes on shores near their source; some tsunamis can cause destruction within hours across an entire ocean basin. Most tsunamis occur in the Pacific region, but they are known to occur in every ocean and sea. Although infrequent, tsunamis are a significant natural hazard with great destructive potential. The 2004 Indonesian tsunami was one of the most deadly disasters in recent years, causing loss of an estimated 229,866 people, including 186,983 dead and 42,883 missing.

1.8.9 Volcanic Eruptions

Volcanic eruptions constitute one of the most dramatic natural disasters. Volcanoes hold a massive reservoir of molten rock (magma) that can vent to the earth's surface. The resulting violent explosion is accompanied by the release of hot gases and materials (pyroclastic flows), lava flows, blasts of superheated steam, and enormous quantities of ash. Ash flows can occur on all sides of the volcano; airborne ash can be dispersed hundreds of miles downwind. Dangerous lava-based mud flows (lahars) and floods also can occur in valleys leading away from volcanoes. The sheer magnitude of the eruptions and the speed with which the explosive blasts and pyroclastic flows occur can make evacuation or escape difficult or impossible.

Volcanic activity is fairly well detectable, in large part because of intensive monitoring. Nevertheless, eruption prediction and warning are among the most challenging endeavors, because of the high levels of uncertainty of the timeframe and event path. This uncertainty leads to challenging decisions about when to evacuate the area because of imminent danger.

According to the USGS, there are at least 30 active volcanoes in the United States that may erupt in the future. These are becoming an increasing concern because of growing population density in volcanic regions, such as those around Mt Rainier, Mt Hood, and Mammoth Lakes. The most recent volcanic disaster in the United States was the eruption of Mount St Helens in Washington State in 1980. This event killed 57 people, impacted more than 200 square miles with ash and debris, caused the largest landslide in recorded history, and cost more than $1.1 billion in timber, civil works, and agricultural losses alone.

1.8.10 Wildfires

In many parts of the world, wild lands have become overgrown with trees and other plant life. When coupled with drought conditions and an ignition source, this buildup of plants can provide the fuel for a potentially disastrous fire. Wildfires often begin unnoticed and can spread with devastating speed, igniting brush, trees, and homes. While some wildfires are caused by lightning strikes, the majority are caused by human activities. These include the use of machinery (eg, sparks from chain saws), discarded smoking materials, poorly tended campfires and burn piles, and arson.

Each year, wildfires damage or destroy thousands of homes and scorch millions of acres. Damage to life and property is largely the consequence of the increased proximity of human settlements to forests and wilderness areas. Shifts in population density and distribution, as well as recreational activities, have placed greater numbers of people, homes, and businesses at risk. In the United States, costs exceed hundreds of millions of dollars annually. In addition to economic losses, injuries and deaths can be attributed to smoke and dust exposure, burns, heat exposure, and exacerbation of chronic medical conditions, as well as to secondary causes such as aircraft and other vehicular crashes.

1.8.11   Winter Storms

A winter storm might include any of the following hazardous conditions: freezing rain, sleet, blizzard conditions with high winds and blowing snow, and below-freezing temperatures. Severe winter storms can cause widespread damage and disruption. Heavy snow often results in paralyzed transportation systems, highway crashes, stranded motorists, and power outages. When accompanied by intense winds, ice, and extreme cold, winter storms can isolate individuals and entire communities.

According to FEMA, between January 2000 and March 2007 there were 21 US Presidential disaster declarations for winter storm activities. According to the National Weather Service, in 2008 there were 21 winter storm–related fatalities and 121 injuries in the United States. The 10-year US average is 47 fatalities per year. Winter storm damages totaled more than $1 billion in 2008.

1.9   INFECTIOUS DISEASE OUTBREAKS

Infectious diseases are caused by pathogenic microorganisms, such as bacteria, viruses, parasites, or fungi. The diseases can be spread, directly or indirectly, from one person to another. Also, many infectious diseases can be transmitted to humans from animals, insects, plants, or contaminated food and water. Infectious diseases are a continuing threat to all persons, regardless of age, gender, lifestyle, ethnic background, and socioeconomic status. Societal, technological, and environmental factors have a dramatic effect on infectious diseases worldwide, facilitating the emergence of new diseases and the reemergence of old ones, sometimes in drug-resistant forms. Environmental changes can affect the incidence of these diseases by altering the habitats and ecology of disease vectors.

Modern demographic and ecological conditions that favor the spread of infectious diseases include rapid population growth; increasing poverty and urban migration; more frequent movement across international boundaries by tourists, workers, immigrants, and refugees; alterations in the habitats of animals and arthropods that transmit disease; increasing numbers of persons with impaired host defenses; and changes in the way that food is processed and distributed. In the globalized world, diseases can spread broadly via international travel and trade. Air travel has increased substantially, and more people are visiting remote locations where they can be exposed to infectious agents that are uncommon in their native countries. A health crisis in one country can impact livelihoods and economies in many parts of the world.

According to the WHO, infectious diseases account for approximately 26% of deaths globally (15 million) and are the leading cause of death in people younger than 50 years.[8] Each year almost 3 million children die of malaria and diarrheal disease alone. Ninety percent of all infectious disease deaths worldwide are caused by six diseases:

➤ Diarrheal disease (eg, due to cholera, dysentery, typhoid fever, and rotavirus gastroenteritis)

➤ Human immunodeficiency virus (HIV) and acquired immunodeficiency syndrome (AIDS)

➤ Malaria

➤ Measles

➤ Pneumonia

➤ Tuberculosis

Certain infectious diseases (eg, diphtheria, tetanus, polio, measles, mumps, rubella, and *Haemophilus influenzae* type b disease) have been virtually eliminated in the United States through universal vaccination, as well as availability of effective medications (eg, antibiotics). Annual immunization remains one of the most important public health strategies for protecting global populations against the spread of seasonal influenza viruses. Ongoing research is needed to develop additional vaccines and more effective treatments to combat infectious diseases that continue to cause serious illness and death worldwide, such as HIV/AIDS, malaria, and tuberculosis.

1.9.1 Foodborne Diseases[9]

In recent years, the United States has experienced several multistate foodborne disease outbreaks, including outbreaks caused by cyclospora parasites on fresh raspberries; hepatitis A virus on frozen strawberries; *Salmonella* bacteria in eggs and peanut butter; and *Escherichia coli* bacteria in apple cider, lettuce, alfalfa

The International Health Regulations

The International Health Regulations (IHR) are an international legal instrument (ie, a 2007 treaty) that is binding on 194 countries across the globe, including all member states of the WHO. The IHR aim to help the global community prevent and respond to acute public health risks that have the potential to cross borders and threaten people worldwide. The IHR also aim to limit interference with global traffic and trade while ensuring public health through the prevention of disease spread.

The IHR require countries to report certain disease outbreaks and public health events to WHO authorities and establish a number of procedures that the WHO must follow to uphold global public health security. The IHR require countries to strengthen existing capacities for public health surveillance and response. The WHO works closely with countries and partners to provide technical guidance and support to mobilize the resources needed to implement the rules in an effective and timely manner. For more information, see http://www.who.int/ihr/en/.

sprouts, and ground beef. The most commonly recognized foodborne infections are caused by the bacteria *Campylobacter*, *Salmonella*, and *E coli* O157:H7 and a group of viruses called *caliciviruses* (also known as Norwalk and Norwalk-like viruses). Many of these outbreaks can be traced to changes in the ways foods are processed, stored, and distributed.

In addition to disease caused by direct microbial contamination, some foodborne diseases are caused by the presence of toxins in the food. For example, the bacterium *Staphylococcus aureus* can grow in some foods and produce a toxin that causes intense vomiting. The rare but deadly disease botulism occurs when the bacterium *Clostridium botulinum* grows and produces a powerful toxin in foods. People also can become ill if a pesticide or other hazardous chemical is added to a food, or if naturally poisonous substances are used to prepare a meal. Every year, people become ill after eating poisonous mushrooms or poisonous reef fishes.

1.9.2   Waterborne Diseases[10]

After a disaster, water-related illnesses can be acquired through a lack of fresh water for good hygiene, lack of sanitation, or increasing insect populations that breed in water and then spread disease. According to the WHO, diarrheal disease accounts for an estimated 4.1% of the total global burden of disease and is responsible for the deaths of 1.8 million people every year.[11] It is estimated that 88% of that burden is attributable to unsafe water supplies and poor sanitation and hygiene and is mostly concentrated in children in developing countries. Waterborne disease can be caused by parasites (eg, schistosomiasis), protozoans (eg, giardiasis, amebiasis), viruses (eg, hepatitis A), and bacteria (eg, cholera, dysentery, typhoid fever).

Milwaukee Cryptosporidium Outbreak

In 1993, the widespread distribution of the *Cryptosporidium* parasite in Milwaukee, Wisconsin, led to the largest waterborne disease outbreak in documented US history. The Howard Avenue water purification plant, one of two water treatment plants serving Milwaukee residents, was contaminated. The primary source of contamination was never officially identified. The high resistance of the cyst form of *Cryptosporidium* to disinfectants such as chlorine enabled it to survive for long periods, while remaining infective.

Over a span of approximately 2 weeks, 403,000 of an estimated 1.61 million Milwaukee-area residents (of whom 880,000 were served by the malfunctioning treatment plant) became ill with the stomach cramps, fever, diarrhea, and dehydration caused by the parasite. More than 100 deaths were attributed to this outbreak, mostly among the elderly and persons with poorly functioning immune systems (such as patients with AIDS); about 4400 people were hospitalized.

1.9.3   Seasonal and Pandemic Influenza

Although influenza (flu) is a common illness each year, many underestimate the potential public health impact of this disease. Yearly influenza causes respiratory illnesses in thousands of individuals, with severe problems usually occurring in children and the elderly, as well as those with chronic disease such as heart and lung disease, diabetes, and illnesses that weaken the immune system.

According to the CDC, every year in the United States about 5% to 20% of the population will get the flu; more than 200,000 will be hospitalized from flu-related complications; and about 36,000 people will die of flu-related causes. If these figures are extrapolated to the rest of the world, there would be about 1 billion cases of flu, about 3 to 5 million cases of severe illness, and 300,000 to 500,000 deaths annually.

Influenza pandemics have occurred at intervals of 10 to 60 years, with three in the 20th century (1918, 1957–1958, and 1967–1968). A pandemic can start when three conditions are met:

➤ A new disease emerges to which a population has little or no immunity.

➤ The disease is infectious for humans.

➤ The disease spreads easily among humans.

For an influenza pandemic to occur, the flu virus must undergo a major change that essentially results in a new form of the virus. This "new" virus will not be recognized by the immune systems of most people, leaving them with little to no natural resistance or immune protection. The large pool of susceptible people

2009 Novel H1N1 Influenza Pandemic

Since April 2009, global attention has been fixed on the emergence and spread of a potentially serious H1N1 influenza A virus throughout the world. As a consequence of confirmed cases of H1N1 disease in four states, on April 26, 2009, the acting secretary of the US Department of Health and Human Services (HHS) declared the existence of a national public health emergency, recognizing that the H1N1 virus had significant potential to affect national security. On June 11, 2009, the WHO raised the pandemic alert level to "Phase 6: Declared Pandemic," signaling that a global pandemic was under way.

With the WHO alert, countries are taking expedient efforts to organize, communicate, and implement planned mitigation measures. As of this writing, it is too early to know how far the virus will spread, how many people will be infected, or how virulent it will become.

For more information about pandemic influenza, refer to http://www.pandemicflu.gov, the official US government Web site on this topic. For global information and updates, refer to the WHO Web site at http://www.who.int.

allows the virus to spread broadly and rapidly, thus creating the potential for a serious public health emergency.

An especially severe influenza pandemic could lead to serious illness and death (even among young and healthy people), social disorder, and economic loss. Everyday life could be disrupted because large numbers of people in many places would become seriously ill at the same time. In 1918, an influenza pandemic killed about 675,000 people in the United States and between 20 and 50 million people around the world. In 2003, the SARS outbreak caused economic losses and social disruption far beyond the affected countries and far out of proportion to the number of cases and deaths. While influenza is distinctly different from SARS, it can be anticipated that a pandemic would have a similarly disruptive effect on societies and economies.

1.10 HUMAN SYSTEMS FAILURES (TECHNOLOGICAL DISASTERS)

Technological disasters can result from hazardous materials spills, structure fires, industrial plant explosions, structural collapses, motor vehicle crashes, train derailments, and breaks in water, gas, or sewer lines. Many of these can be attributed to unintentional human systems failures, such as poorly designed buildings or flawed equipment, and human errors due to inadequate training, worker distraction, or fatigue. In these disasters, workers, area residents, and responders may be at risk from exposures to contaminated air, water, food, fires, and explosions, as well as hazardous materials (eg, chemical, biologic, or radioactive) released into the environment.

1.10.1   Human Stampede and Crowd Surges

Crowd surges are true "mass casualty incidents." Triggers of human stampede include fires and evacuations, as well as crowd surges at sporting events (notably soccer matches), concerts, festivals, religious pilgrimages, and retail sales and giveaway events. In most cases, casualties and fatalities occur as a result of traumatic injuries and asphyxiation from crushing and trampling, as well as from burns and smoke inhalation (as a result of structure fires). Further hampering scene management of these disasters are the confusion, panic, and logistical complexities of mass gatherings. Recent examples include the following:

➤ May 2002: 30 injured at rapper Eminem's concert in Washington, DC

➤ February 2003: 21 dead in Chicago from a nightclub stampede

➤ January 2005: 265 people killed as Hindu pilgrims stampede near a remote temple in Maharashtra, India

➤ August 2005: 1000 people killed in a Baghdad bridge stampede

➤ November 2007: three people killed and more than 30 injured at the Supermarket Carrefour in Chongqing, China, when the shop was offering 20% discounts on cooking oil

➤ September 2008: 147 people killed at the Chamunda Devi temple in Jodhpur, India; the tragedy may have been triggered by a rumor that a bomb was planted in the temple complex

1.10.2   Industrial Disasters

Major industrial incidents typically involve the release of hazardous materials such as oil and gas products, radioactive materials, and other potentially harmful chemicals. They can result in numerous fatalities and countless more injuries, pose the risk of widespread contamination, and trigger secondary incidents, such as explosions and fires. In addition, they often exact a heavy toll on local communities in terms of lives lost, jobs lost, and prolonged emotional recovery. Public health emergencies can arise from significant long-term environmental contamination such as occurred in the 1984 Union Carbide pesticide plant tragedy in Bhopal, India, and the 1986 Chernobyl nuclear power plant meltdown.

Data on the release of hazardous materials from industrial sites are limited. In the United States, the Agency for Toxic Substances and Disease Registry has maintained a state-based Hazardous Substances Emergency Events Surveillance (HSEES) system since 1990. In 2005, a total of 8603 events involving the acute release of hazardous materials were reported by the 15 states that participate in the HSEES system.[12] The most commonly reported categories of substances were "other inorganic substances" (which excludes chemicals in the categories of acids, bases, ammonia, and chlorine), volatile organic compounds, and mixtures involving substances from different categories that were mixed or formed from a reaction before release. In 2005, 778 events (9.0% of all reported events) resulted in 2034 injuries and 69 deaths (3.4%). The most frequently reported injuries were respiratory irritation, headaches, and dizziness/central nervous system symptoms. Facility evacuations were ordered for 481 events (5.6%).

1.10.3   Structure Collapse

Building and other structure collapses occur infrequently in the United States. The most famous event not related to terrorism was the walkway collapse of

Minneapolis Bridge Collapse

The I-35W Mississippi River bridge was an eight-lane steel bridge that carried Interstate 35W across the Mississippi River in Minneapolis, Minnesota. The bridge is noteworthy because, during the evening rush hour on August 1, 2007, it collapsed into the river and onto the riverbanks beneath, killing 13 people and injuring 145 others. The bridge carried almost 140,000 vehicles daily.

Immediately after the collapse, help arrived from the multiple regional emergency response personnel, charities, and volunteers. Only a few vehicles were submerged, but many people were stranded on the collapsed sections of the bridge. Several vehicles caught fire, including a semi-trailer truck. A school bus carrying 60 children ended up resting dangerously against the guardrail of the collapsed structure, near the burning truck. Triage centers at the ends of the bridge routed 50 victims to area hospitals, some in trucks, as ambulances were in short supply. Many of the injured had blunt trauma injuries. During the first 40 hours, 11 area hospitals treated 98 victims, including at least 22 children.

On November 13, 2008, the National Transportation Safety Board (NTSB) cited a design flaw (ie, undersized gusset plates) as the likely cause of the collapse and asserted that additional weight on the bridge at the time of the collapse contributed to the failure. The NTSB determined that corrosion was not a significant factor.

the Hyatt Regency Hotel in Kansas City, Missouri, on July 17, 1981. One hundred eleven people were killed and hundreds more were injured in this, the greatest intrinsic structural failure in US history. The collapse was traced to engineering failures and shortcuts taken during construction. The resulting civil lawsuits cost billions of dollars and far exceeded the cost of the building itself. More recent examples include the November 2003 collapse of a gangway leading to the Queen Mary II in France, which killed 16 people; a second-story balcony collapse in Chicago, which killed 12 people on June 29, 2003; and the 2007 collapse of a large bridge in Minneapolis, which killed 13 people.

Structure collapses also result from earthquakes or other natural disasters. These types of disasters also pose a significant risk of explosions, chemical exposures, and other secondary hazards.

1.10.4 Structure Fires

Most fires occur in residential structures and generate limited numbers of casualties. However, the potential for large numbers of casualties from high-rise building fires must be considered. In 2008, there were an estimated 515,000 structure fires in the United States, resulting in 2900 deaths and 14,960 injuries. Economic losses exceeded $12.3 billion.[13] The collapse of the World Trade Center in New York City on September 11, 2001, has increased attention to the prevention of all structure fires, and particularly high-rise building fires and high-rise firefighting tactics. The most common causes of fire-related injury and death include carbon monoxide poisoning, burns, smoke inhalation, heat stress, and inhalation of toxic gases, as well as traumatic injuries and exacerbation of chronic medical conditions. In a fire, children, elderly adults, and disabled persons are at increased risk of injury and death. Firefighters also are at risk of harm. In addition to the structure fire itself, the very real possibility of secondary hazards must be considered, including exposure to hazardous materials and structural collapse.

1.10.5 Transportation Disasters

Transportation ranks far and away as the most common technological health hazard. In 2007, 41,059 people were killed in the estimated 6,024,000 police-reported motor vehicle traffic crashes in the United States; 2,491,000 people were injured.[14] In addition to roadway incidents, serious injuries and deaths occur each year from travel by air, rail, and water. Transportation disasters also involve secondary hazards, including explosions, fires, and release of hazardous materials.

Washington, DC, Train Collision

On June 22, 2009, a Metro transit train smashed into the rear of another at the height of the capital city's Monday evening rush hour, killing nine people and injuring scores of others as the front end of the trailing train jackknifed violently into the air and fell atop the first. Cars of both trains were ripped open and smashed together in the worst accident in the Metrorail system's 33-year history. Rescue workers treated 76 people at the scene and sent some of them to local hospitals, six with critical injuries. The impact of the crash was so powerful that the striking train was compressed to about one-third of its original size. Investigators are determining whether operator error may have contributed to this tragic event.

1.11   CONFLICT-BASED DISASTERS

These disasters are intentional, human-caused events and include war, civil disorder and political violence, and terrorism. War and civil disorder generate complex humanitarian emergencies characterized by social, political, economic, and other factors that often provoke population displacement as either internally displaced populations or refugees. Such events are accompanied by a deterioration of living conditions and public health support systems.

Major conflict-based disasters represent a critical threat to the health, safety, security, and well-being of entire communities and countries, affecting large groups of people. In these situations, the proportion of indirect deaths is usually much higher (70% to 90%) than that of direct deaths, secondary to diminished access to and availability of care, food, potable water, sanitation, and housing. Recent examples of conflict-based disasters include the Sri Lankan civil war, Israeli-Palestinian conflict, Afghan civil war, Darfur conflict, and Iraq war.

Darfur Conflict in Sudan

Africa's biggest country, Sudan, is divided along lines of religion, ethnicity, tribe, and economic activity (ie, nomadic and sedentary). The country has been in near-constant war since its independence in 1956. The current conflict in Darfur is complex, caused by a host of political, social, economic, and environmental problems. The result is a humanitarian crisis affecting millions of people.

International relief organizations are working to help meet the most basic needs of affected populations, including food, shelter, water, and sanitation facilities. In May 2005, the CRED published an analysis of mortality in Darfur. Their estimate stated that from September 2003 to January 2005, between 98,000 and 181,000 persons had died in Darfur, including 63,000 to 146,000 excess deaths.

1.11.1 Civil Disturbance

Civil disturbances are increasing worldwide as populations merge, migration occurs, and competition for resources becomes more dominant. Civil unrest can occur whenever a group feels that some aspect of society is antithetic or apathetic to their views, rights, or needs. Examples include labor strikes, sit-ins, large demonstrations, and parades, which can escalate into chaos, riots, and sabotage. If public safety is at risk, law enforcement personnel may use tear gas, pepper spray, or other less lethal weapons (eg, Tasers™, "bean bag" munitions) to control and disperse unruly crowds. These devices are designed to incapacitate persons without causing serious harm. These events can result in significant numbers of casualties and tax the health system to care for them. Disruption of local infrastructure also may occur during very severe events. Public utilities such as water, fuel, and electricity, as well as public infrastructure for communication, may be temporarily unavailable.

1.11.2 Terrorism

Terrorism is a broad term that describes the use of force or violence against persons or property for purposes of intimidation, coercion, or ransom. Terrorist threats can come from many sources and take many forms. Recent attention has focused on terrorist use of toxic or poisonous chemicals, infectious disease organisms, radioactive materials, explosive incendiary or poison gas bombs, grenades, rockets or missiles, and landmines or similar devices, but explosives and firearms are the most commonly used tools of terrorists. During the initial assessment of any mass casualty situation, emergency responders must evaluate the possibility that it could be the result of terrorism.

Terrorists often use threats to create fear among the public—to try to convince citizens that their government is powerless to prevent terrorism, and to get immediate publicity for their causes. This could include threats of mass destruction or more traditional kidnappings and airplane hijackings in which hostages are held in exchange for money or some other demand. In recent years, public awareness of the threat of terrorism in the United States has grown dramatically.

The annual global terror reports from the US State Department regularly list bombs as responsible for about 75% of all terror events worldwide and firearms for almost all the rest. On April 20, 1999, two students entered Columbine High School in Columbine, Colorado, began shooting students and teachers at random, and eventually killed themselves, but not before killing 12 of their classmates and one teacher. On September 1, 2004, Chechan separatists lay siege to the Beslan School Number One (Beslan, Russia), taking more than 1100 students and teachers hostage, including 777 children. They rigged the building with improvised explosives and threatened to detonate them if their demands for an end to the Second Chechan War were not met. On day 3 of the standoff, Russian forces attempted to rescue the hostages, but the ensuing battle left 334 hostages (including 186 children) dead and hundreds injured. On April 16, 2007, a student opened fire on helpless classmates at Virginia Polytechnic Institute and State University (Virginia Tech) in Blacksburg, Virginia, killing 32 and wounding many others before committing suicide. These events demonstrate the potential of terrorists to create significant mass casualty events through the use of firearms and explosives, the most commonly used methods of terrorism.

The potential for an individual or group to deliberately contaminate food, water, and other consumer products is real and cannot be ignored. Crops, livestock, processing and distribution chains, storage facilities, and transport modes all provide potential venues for overt and covert forms of terrorism. Even the threat or suggestion of contamination could be sufficient to seriously disrupt the economies and lifestyles of targeted populations. Government response plans have focused on developing resources in local, state, and federal government agencies, including health departments, emergency responders (eg, police and fire departments, hazardous materials [HAZMAT] units, and emergency medical systems), and federal and military response units. Education and training efforts have been directed to better prepare citizens and health professionals for terrorism.

Selected Forms of Terrorism

Terrorism includes the use of chemical, biologic, radiologic, nuclear, and explosive agents. Deaths are typically direct, although indirect morbidity due to psychological trauma is significant.

Chemical terrorism includes the use of chemical agents such as the nerve agent sarin, vesicants such as mustard, and inhalants such as phosgene. Terrorists could also cause the release of industrial chemicals such as chlorine, ammonia, or other agents used in manufacturing and transported via truck and rail.

Bioterrorism is the use of a living organism such as a virus or bacteria (or its products) against a civilian population to coerce, intimidate, or cause panic. The CDC categorizes bioterrorism agents on the basis of the potential threat of these agents. These are designated by the CDC as category A, B, or C agents, in which category A agents are considered the highest health security priority. The category A agents include *Bacillus anthracis* (the cause of anthrax), the smallpox virus, *Clostridium botulinum* toxin (the cause of botulism), viral hemorrhagic fever viruses, *Yesinia pestis* (the cause of plague), and *Francisella tularensis* (the cause of tularemia).

Radiological terrorism is the use of radioactive materials to enact terrorism. It usually refers to an intentional "dirty" bomb release, which is an explosive laced with a radioactive material such as cesium 137. Most deaths are attributable to the explosive used rather than radiation exposure, but the desired effect of such an attack would be to induce panic and fear due to the spreading of radioactive material.

Nuclear terrorism refers to the intentional detonation of nuclear weapons. The destruction of entire cities is possible, with the number of burn casualties and radiation injuries resulting from such weapons being staggering.

Use of explosives by terrorists generally refers to homicide and suicide bombings and the detonation of intentional explosive devices. This form of terrorism is the most likely and is on the rise. Most deaths are attributable to direct traumatic injuries.

The impact of terrorism can vary considerably from injuries and loss of life to property damage and disruptions in services such as electricity, water supply, public transportation, and communications. Long-term consequences involve costly environmental cleanup and prolonged public anxiety. In all forms of terrorism, whether involving biologic weapons, toxic chemicals, or conventional explosives, local health professionals will provide acute and follow-up care to affected individuals and communities.

A critical component in dealing with terrorism and other disasters is a strong public health infrastructure. Investment in public health systems will enhance the capacity to detect and contain rare or unusual disease outbreaks, whether deliberately induced or naturally occurring. Establishing more effective strategies against bioterrorism, for example, has the additional benefit of improving response to natural epidemics and new or emerging diseases. Capacities needed to cope effectively with the consequences of an act of bioterrorism can build on the systems used to respond to natural disease outbreaks. This allows for a dual-use response infrastructure that improves the ability of health professionals and health agencies to respond to multiple hazards while taking into account the unique and complex challenges presented by terrorism.

1.12 CORE CONCEPTS IN DISASTER MANAGEMENT

Disaster management aims to minimize, or avoid, the potential losses from hazards, assure prompt and appropriate assistance to affected populations, and achieve rapid and effective recovery. Disaster management is an ongoing process, involving the following 4 activities, by which governments, businesses, and communities plan for and reduce the impact of disasters:

➤ *Mitigation* – Minimizing the likelihood of disaster occurrence (eg, building codes and zoning);

➤ *Preparedness* – Planning how to respond (eg, exercises/drills; education and training; advance warning systems);

➤ *Response* – Efforts to protect public health, safety, and security and minimize economic and environmental losses (eg, search and rescue; disaster relief); and

➤ *Recovery* – Returning the community to normal (eg, temporary housing; grant support; medical care).

1.12.1 Mitigation

The mitigation phase, and indeed the whole disaster management cycle, includes the shaping of public policies and plans that either modify the causes of disasters or minimize their impact on people, property, and infrastructure. Mitigation efforts seek to eliminate or reduce the probability of disaster occurrence, or reduce the effects of unavoidable events. The effectiveness of such efforts depends on the availability of accurate information on potential hazards and appropriate countermeasures that can be taken to prevent or limit damage. Disaster mitigation involves building codes; zoning and land use management; engineering; building use regulations and safety codes; preventive health care; and public education. Examples include earthquake-proofing of buildings, installation of sprinkler systems to suppress fires, pharmaceutical stockpiling, and development of alternate care sites for prolonged public health emergencies.

1.12.2   Preparedness

The goal of disaster preparedness is to achieve a satisfactory level of readiness to respond to any disaster situation through measures that strengthen the technical and managerial capacity of governments, organizations, and communities. During the preparedness phase, government officials, business leaders, and other individuals develop policies and procedures to save lives, minimize disaster damage, and enhance disaster response operations. The preparedness process is directly dependent on the strength of pre-event preparation. As shown in (Figure 1-3), this involves a continuous cycle of planning, organizing/equipping, training, exercising, and evaluating, and improving.

Preparedness measures include disaster planning; public and professional education and training; disaster exercises and drills; early warning systems; emergency information dissemination and communication systems; evacuation procedures; resource inventories; emergency personnel/contact lists; and mutual aid agreements. The effectiveness of preparedness depends on knowledge of potential hazards and appropriate countermeasures, as well as the extent to

FIGURE 1-3

The Disaster Preparedness Cycle

Source: http://www.fema
.gov/emergency/nims/
Preparedness.shtm.

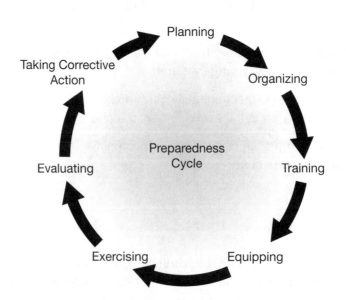

The PRE–DISASTER Paradigm™

For the NDLS Program, the PRE–DISASTER Paradigm was developed to reinforce key elements for enhancing personal and community preparedness. The mnemonic encompasses:

➤ *Planning and practice*

➤ *Resilience*

➤ *Education*

Planning and practice. The strength of preparedness depends on careful and ongoing planning, as well as continual practicing of those plans. Planning includes the design, implementation, and ongoing evaluation of efforts to help communities, institutions, and individuals prepare for, respond to, and recover from disasters and public health emergencies. Effective planning requires integrated collaboration from the entire disaster response system to include emergency management and public safety agencies, local public health agencies, hospitals (both private and public), local clinics, emergency medical services (both private and public), businesses, and community groups. Contingencies also must be considered (eg, to address scarcity of resources). The strength of preparedness depends on careful and ongoing planning, as well as continual practicing and evaluation of those plans.

Resilience. Being prepared (through planning, education, and training) can reduce fear, anxiety, and losses associated with a disaster and build resiliency. Resilience is the ability of individuals and communities to rebound to a reasonable state of normalcy after exposure to disasters, serious emergencies, and other traumatic, tragic, and stressful events (such as family and relationship problems, serious health problems, or workplace and financial stressors). In advance of a disaster, resilience can be built into a community by educating the population about local disaster planning and response efforts and assisting them with the development of personal and family preparedness plans.

Being resilient does not mean that a person does not experience difficulty or distress. Emotional pain and sadness are common in people who have suffered major adversity or trauma in their lives. Resilience is not a trait that people either have or do not have. It involves behaviors, thoughts, and actions that can be learned and developed in anyone. Resilience also refers to plans that return the infrastructure of a community back to normal as soon as possible after an event.

Education. Education is paramount and critical to preparedness. All responders, regardless of specialty or area of expertise, require a fundamental, basic level of education and training in all-hazards disaster management and disaster life support. They must understand their role and how it is integrated with other segments of the disaster response system. Effective education programs can help minimize the impact of a disaster as well as build resiliency. For example, education about the warning signs of a tornado or hurricane can save lives by empowering people to take appropriate protective action.

The development and dissemination of comprehensive curricula to train all potential health system responders for disasters and public health emergencies (such as through the NDLS Program) presents a daunting challenge. That is because disasters, terrorism, and public health emergencies can occur in multiple scenarios, with diverse clinical and public health outcomes, many of which are not addressed in current health professional school or continuing education programs. Certainly, the topic areas that need to be learned by all potential health system responders must be relevant to the roles they will play and be reasonably attainable, considering time and financial resources.

The elements of the PRE–DISASTER Paradigm are discussed and reinforced in Chapters 2 and 3 of this manual.

which government agencies, nongovernmental organizations, and the general public are able to make use of this information in an emergency.

1.12.3   Response

Once a disaster occurs, the response phase involves implementation of personal, community, and facility disaster plans. Community response plans will be implemented through a local incident management structure, which may be scaled according to the disaster situation. The aim of disaster response is to provide immediate assistance to protect lives, preserve health, and support the morale of affected populations. Assistance may range from providing specific but limited aid, such as assisting evacuees with transport, temporary shelter, and food, to establishing semi-permanent settlement in camps and other locations. Response also may involve initial repairs to damaged infrastructure. The focus in the response phase is on meeting the basic needs of affected people until more permanent and sustainable solutions can be found.

During a disaster, myriad public and private sector agencies are often called upon to deal with immediate response and recovery. To be able to respond effectively, their efforts must be integrated at all levels, which involves experienced leaders, trained personnel, adequate transport and logistic support, appropriate communications, and standard operating procedures for working in disaster situations. Federal, state, and local government agencies have unmatched resources and legal authority to address disaster-related needs. Government authorities will coordinate extensive logistical efforts, such as moving large amounts of relief supplies. Humanitarian organizations are often strongly present in this phase of the disaster management cycle.

1.12.4   Recovery

Recovery is the final and usually longest phase of the disaster management cycle. Recovery begins immediately after an event has occurred, as affected populations begin to restore their lives and the infrastructure that supports them. There is no distinct point at which disaster relief changes into recovery and then into long-term sustainable development. Recovery can be enhanced through the building of personal and community resilience during the disaster preparedness phase. By addressing and prioritizing short- and long-term recovery measures in advance, affected communities may avoid excess morbidity and mortality in a serious disaster or public health emergency.

Recovery activities continue until all systems return to normal or better. Recovery measures, both short and long term, include returning vital life-support systems

The DISASTER Paradigm™

For the NDLS Program, a useful mnemonic, called the DISASTER Paradigm™, is used to identify the key elements of disaster response and recovery:

➤ *Detection*

➤ *Incident management*

➤ *Safety and security*

➤ *Assess hazards*

➤ *Support*

➤ *Triage and treatment*

➤ *Evacuation*

➤ *Recovery*

The DISASTER Paradigm is a practical learning tool that is incorporated into all NDLS courses to enhance communication consistency among disaster response personnel and agencies. Use of the DISASTER Paradigm can benefit all responders by helping them answer the question: "Do my needs exceed my resources?" As defined at the beginning of this chapter, this is a critical question in disaster life support. The DISASTER Paradigm is covered in greater depth in Chapter 6 of this manual.

to minimal operating standards; temporary housing; public information; health and safety education; reconstruction; counseling programs; and impact studies. Information resources and services include data collection related to rebuilding, and documentation of lessons learned. A critical element in community recovery is reestablishing public health and healthcare infrastructures and ensuring access to preventive, curative, and rehabilitative programs and services. There will be many opportunities during the recovery period to enhance prevention and increase preparedness, thus reducing vulnerability to future events.

1.13 DISASTERS AND PUBLIC HEALTH

The public health implications of disasters can be widespread and variable, depending on many factors including the nature, scale, and time of the event; level of preparedness; and response capacity.

1.13.1   Biologic Events

Human exposure to biologic agents may occur through inhalation, skin (cutaneous) exposure, or ingestion of contaminated food or water. In recent years, global concern has increased about bioterrorism, the deliberate use of certain pathogens or biologic products by terrorists to influence the conduct of government or to intimidate or coerce a civilian population. As was learned in the spring of 2003, epidemics resulting from emerging infectious diseases like SARS can cause widespread civil panic and conditions similar to a bioterrorist event.

Effective response to a disease outbreak (natural or intended) depends on rapid identification of the causative agent and specific diagnosis. To enhance detection and treatment capabilities, health professionals should be familiar with the clinical manifestations, diagnostic techniques, isolation precautions, treatment, and prophylaxis for likely causative agents (eg, smallpox, pneumonic plague, anthrax, viral hemorrhagic fevers). For some of these agents, delay in the health system response could result in a potentially devastating number of casualties. To mitigate such consequences, early identification and intervention are imperative. Front-line health professionals must have an increased level of suspicion regarding the possible intentional use of biologic agents as well as an increased sensitivity to reporting those suspicions to public health authorities, who, in turn, must be willing to evaluate a predictable increase in false-positive reports. Clinicians should report noticeable increases in unusual illnesses, symptom complexes, or disease patterns (even without definitive diagnosis) to public health authorities. Prompt reporting of unusual patterns of illness can allow public health officials to initiate an epidemiologic investigation earlier than would be possible if the report awaited definitive etiologic diagnosis.

Health system response efforts require coordination and planning with emergency management agencies, law enforcement, health care facilities, and social service agencies. Public health agencies should ensure that physicians and other health professionals know who to call with reports of suspicious cases and clusters of infectious diseases, and should work to build a good relationship with the local medical community. Resource integration is absolutely necessary to establish adequate capacity to initiate rapid investigation of an outbreak, to educate the public, to begin mass distribution of medications and vaccines, to ensure mass medical care, and to control public anger and fear.

1.13.2   Chemical Emergencies

Release of chemical agents can occur via unintended or deliberate means, such as through a spill from a damaged railroad tank car or an explosion at an industrial facility with resultant contamination of air, food, water, or consumer products. Concern has increased about potential terrorist attacks involving the use of toxic chemical agents to cause widespread panic and harm. Chemicals could be released as bombs, sprayed from aircraft and boats, or disseminated by other means to intentionally create a hazard to people and the environment.

Health effects of chemical agents range from irritation and burning of eyes, skin, and mucous membranes to rapid cardiopulmonary collapse and death. Such effects are usually immediate (a few seconds) or very rarely delayed (several hours to days). Immediate symptoms of exposure to chemical agents may include blurred vision, eye irritation, difficulty breathing, and nausea. Affected persons may require urgent medical attention. Several persons presenting with the same symptoms should alert clinicians and hospital staff to the possibility of a chemical attack. If an attack occurs, most victims will likely arrive at the hospital within a short time period. This situation differentiates a chemical attack from a biologic attack involving infectious microorganisms, in which time elapses between exposure and the development of symptoms.

Some, but not all, chemical agents have a high potential for secondary contamination from victims to responders. Most exposures to true vapors—as opposed to suspended mists or aerosols—generate exposure but not contamination. This requires that medical treatment facilities have clearly defined procedures for handling contaminated casualties, many of whom will transport themselves to the facility. Precautions must be used until thorough decontamination has been performed or the specific chemical agent is identified. Health professionals must

The Sarin Attack on the Tokyo Subway

On Monday March 20, 1995, five members of a Japan-based religious group, Aum Shinrikyo, entered the Tokyo Subway at the peak of the morning rush hour carrying plastic bags of liquid sarin nerve agent. Each of the perpetrators began to place the bags wrapped in newspaper on the floor of the subway car and puncture the bags with sharpened umbrella tips as they exited the train cars. The resulting vapors from the sarin sickened over 5,000 and killed a dozen. Six-hundred and eighty-eight (688) victims were transported to hospitals via EMS, while the majority (88%) were transported to hospitals via other means. No decontamination was performed for the majority of victims either on the scene or at the hospitals. Because of the lack of decontamination, approximately 10% of emergency medical services (EMS) responders and 23% of staff at the major receiving hospital developed symptoms of secondary intoxication. Once victims of vapor exposure were instructed to remove their clothing—no more healthcare workers were affected. Antidotes were in short supply and were redistributed from rural areas that had stocked antidotes for the treatment of pesticide poisoning.

Lessons Learned:

➤ Chemical attacks by terrorist are possible and must be considered in planning

➤ Most victims from acute event disasters will self-transport to the hospital

➤ Contaminated victims will arrive at the hospital and hospitals must plan accordingly

➤ For vapor exposures—removing the clothing will prevent exposure via off-gassing to health care providers

➤ Communities must insure adequate supplies of critical antidotes for treating chemical event casualties

first protect themselves (eg, by using protective suits, respiratory protection, and chemical-resistant gloves) because secondary contamination with even small amounts of these substances (particularly nerve agents such as VX) can be lethal.

Efficient deployment of hazardous materials (HAZMAT) teams and other personnel trained in decontamination procedures is critical to control a chemical agent attack. Although all major cities and emergency medical systems have plans and equipment in place to address this situation, health professionals must be aware of principles involved in managing persons exposed to these agents. Health professionals and other responders also need quick access to current information on preparing for a chemical emergency, handling contaminated persons, hazard recognition and assessment, health effects, and accessing emergency assistance. With adequate resources and planning, health professionals and the public can better prepare themselves to recognize an emergency situation and react effectively to protect themselves and others from harm.

1.13.3   Radiation Emergencies

A radiation emergency involves the release of potentially dangerous radioactive materials into the environment. Such incidents can occur anywhere radioactive isotopes are used, stored, or transported. Radiation provokes a special fear, but, with appropriate understanding and preparation, effective clinical care can be provided to exposed people. Radiation can be easily detected with equipment carried by many emergency responders. Radioactive materials may contaminate homes, workplaces, and other resources, requiring extensive and costly remediation and the potential disruption of lives and livelihoods for long periods of time. Serious psychological problems can result in those who think they are being, or have been, exposed.

In the event of a terrorist attack or other radiation disaster, clinicians will play vital roles as responders and as sources of accurate information for affected individuals and communities. The immediate clinical effects of large doses of radiation are well known and can be assessed with the use of simple laboratory tests such as blood cell counts. To decrease morbidity and mortality from a radiation disaster or terrorist attack, health professionals should have a basic understanding of radiation illness and treatment principles. Radiation exerts its toxic effect on biologic systems through ionization, which creates tissue damage by the generation of free radicals, disruption of chemical bonds, and direct damage to cellular DNA and enzymes.

Optimal management of radiation casualties requires:

➤ Knowledge of the type and dose of radiation received

➤ Recognition of the manifestations of radiation sickness

➤ Use of standard medical care

➤ Decontamination

➤ Decorporation techniques

The health effects of radiation exposure tend to be directly proportional to the amount of radiation absorbed by the body (radiation dose) and are determined by the:

➤ Radiation type (ie, alpha, beta, X-ray, or gamma radiation)

➤ Means of exposure, internal or external (absorbed by the skin, inhaled, or ingested)

➤ Duration of exposure

Externally contaminated individuals may expose or contaminate others with whom they come in close contact and should avoid such contact until they have been appropriately decontaminated. The health threat to response personnel is low, however, and can be minimized by using universal safety precautions (mask, gown, gloves). Persons who have inhaled or ingested radioactive material require medical attention. Currently, there are no reliable antidotes to treat exposed persons once radiation has been inhaled or ingested, but symptoms can be treated effectively. Oral and intravenous agents are available that can help remove certain radioactive materials from the body.

Goiania, Brazil, Radiation Emergency

In 1985, a private radiotherapy institute in Goiania, Brazil, moved to a new location, leaving behind an unsecured cesium 137 radiotherapy unit that had previously been used in cancer therapy. The source remained in the vacant building for about 2 years. It was discovered by two persons who entered the premises and, not knowing what the unit was but thinking it might have some scrap value, removed the radioactive cesium 137 source assembly. They took the assembly home, and when they attempted to dismantle it, the source capsule ruptured, exposing them to radiation. This resulted in localized burns to their bodies; one of the men later had to have an arm amputated. The radioactive source was in the form of cesium chloride salt, which is highly soluble and readily dispersible. As a consequence, they contaminated themselves, hundreds of others, and the surrounding city and environment. Thus began one of the most serious radiation incidents ever to have occurred.

A local physicist was the first to assess the scale of the incident and took actions on his own initiative to evacuate two areas. After appropriate authorities were informed, several other sites of significant contamination were quickly identified and secured. Many individuals incurred external and internal exposure. In total, some 112,000 persons were monitored, of whom 249 were contaminated either internally or externally. Four deaths were attributed to this exposure. Some exposed persons suffered very high internal and external contamination owing to the way they handled the cesium chloride powder, such as eating with contaminated hands and via contamination of buildings, furnishings, and utensils.

1.13.4   Bombings and Explosions

Explosions can occur accidentally or as a result of a conflict or terrorism. Across the globe, the threat of terrorism involving the use of explosive agents in urban or otherwise crowded environments has become a reality. Increasing population density and urbanization, coupled with the ubiquity of large buildings, mass transit, and mass gatherings, create the potential for a serious disaster involving multiple casualties.

Bombings are blatant and emphatic and, by their very nature, gain immediate public attention. Explosive events are inherently unpredictable. Despite widespread concerns regarding biologic and chemical attacks, conventional explosives are the most commonly used terrorist weapons because they are the easiest to create, obtain, and use. The medical consequences of the detonation of a conventional explosive include death and acute injury, as well as destruction of critical infrastructure such as buildings, roads, and utilities. Health care needs include immediate emergency trauma care, follow-up medical and surgical care, forensic disposition of bodies and body parts, and mental health care.

Mass trauma related to explosions can produce unique patterns of injury that are seldom seen outside of military hospitals.[15] When explosions occur, they have the potential to inflict multiorgan, life-threatening injuries on many victims simultaneously. The impact of an explosive event depends largely on the composition and amount of explosive materials involved, the surrounding environment, delivery method (if a bomb), distance between the victim and the blast, and any intervening protective barriers or environmental hazards. Blast-related injuries can present unique triage, diagnostic, and management challenges to physicians and other health professionals. First responders run the risk of being caught by subsequent explosions specifically timed to target them, called *secondary devices*.

After an explosive event, health professionals and hospitals must be prepared to treat scores or hundreds of casualties. Their response, however, may be

Terrorist Bombings in Mumbai, India

In 2008, a terrorist attack involved more than 10 coordinated shootings and bombings across Mumbai, India's financial capital and largest city. The attacks began on November 26 and lasted until November 29, 2008. Indian and US authorities linked the attacks to militants inside Pakistan. At least 164 victims (civilians and security personnel) and nine attackers were killed. Among the dead were 28 foreign nationals from 10 countries. At least 308 persons were injured. International reaction to the attacks was widespread, with many countries and international organizations condemning the attacks and expressing their condolences and assistance to the government of India and the civilian victims.

complicated by the loss of utilities (eg, electricity, water), difficulty in transporting victims, lack of trained personnel, and damage to the hospital infrastructure. Similar effects can be encountered in natural disasters such as tornadoes, earthquakes, and industrial or gas main explosions.

1.13.5 Disasters and Mental Health

Experiencing a disaster can be one of the most serious traumatic events a person can endure, which can have both short- and long-term effects. Most people who experience a disaster, whether as a victim or responder, will have some form of psychological, physical, cognitive, behavioral and/or emotional response to the event. All of these can be normal responses to a witnessed traumatic event.

Disaster events that seem to have the most significant behavioral and mental health impact are those that:

➤ Occur with little or no warning;

➤ Pose a serious threat to personal safety;

➤ Create fear of the unknown or delayed health effects;

➤ Occur with uncertain duration; and

➤ Result from malicious intent (eg, terrorism, which has an overriding objective to inflict psychological pain, trauma, anxiety, and panic).

Post-disaster responses are wide-ranging, from mild stress responses to more serious post-traumatic stress disorder (PTSD), major depression, or acute stress disorder. Although acute stress disorder and PTSD receive the most publicity following disasters, the majority of affected persons, including those referred to as the "well but worried," have somatic symptoms below the threshold of a diagnosable psychiatric disorder. Ideally, all affected populations will be supported by a coordinated system of family and community health resources, as well as local primary care and psychological services.

1.13.6 Health Implications of Climate Change

Significant advances have occurred in the understanding of global climate change, and a large volume of published literature on this topic has appeared, particularly in the last half-century. The Intergovernmental Panel on Climate Change, other scientific bodies, and researchers assert that changes in the climate system are occurring, and is evident from observations of increases in global average air and ocean temperatures, widespread melting of snow and ice, and rising global average sea level.[16-18] Though the cause of climate change continues to be debated (eg, greenhouse gas emissions vs. planetary cycle), scientific consensus is growing that climate change is occurring and at a greater rate than previously predicted. The potential linkages between climate change and evolving disaster risk trends and patterns are complex and continue to be debated.

Health effects most commonly predicted are related to heat waves, climate events related to changes in water levels (either extreme flooding or droughts), and increases in infectious and vector-borne diseases. Additional modeling has been conducted to estimate more indirect health effects of global climate change, including the impact of changes in food yields and water supplies on nutrition and hydration. The effects of climate change may be widespread, with impacts on ecosystems, land composition, sea levels, weather patterns, and ice coverage. The potential for such effects requires continued attention from all health professionals.

1.14 SUMMARY

This chapter defines the essential terminology necessary for those involved in the health response to disasters. It presents the current classification of disasters into three distinct categories: natural, human system failure (technological), and conflict based. The chapter discusses the 4 phases of disaster management: mitigation, preparedness, response, and recovery. It introduces the PRE-DISASTER Paradigm as a useful mnemonic for remembering key components of disaster preparedness (ie, planning and practice, resilience, and education). It also introduces the DISASTER Paradigm (detection, incident command, safety and security, assess hazards, support, triage and treatment, evacuation, and recovery) as a learning tool for remembering key aspects of disaster response and recovery.

Global trends indicate that the frequency and magnitude of—and, thus, the risk of exposure to—potential disaster hazards is on the rise. All health professionals need to become proficient in the recognition, diagnosis, and treatment of mass casualties under an all-hazards approach to disaster management. Health professionals are on the front lines when dealing with injury and disease, whether caused by microbes, environmental hazards, natural disasters, highway collisions, terrorism, or other calamities. Early detection and reporting are critical to minimize casualties through astute teamwork by public- and private-sector health and emergency response personnel.

The best way to make homes and communities safer is to be prepared before disaster strikes. Preparedness can be achieved through thoughtful planning and can ensure that if a disaster occurs, people are ready to get through it safely and respond to it effectively. Preparedness reinforces the need for constant vigilance and planning to prepare for and respond to new and unexpected public health threats.

1.15 SELF-LEARNING SCENARIOS

After completing the CDLS® course and each of the chapters in this manual, take time to work through the 4 scenarios presented in Appendix A. The scenarios are designed for the application and reinforcement of "core" concepts and principles in disaster life support.

REFERENCES

1. Task Force on Quality Control of Disaster Management/World Association of Disaster and Emergency Medicine. Glossary of terms. In: Health Disaster Management: Guidelines for Evaluation and Research in the Utstein Style. *Prehosp Disast Med.* 2002;17(suppl 3): 144–167.

2. Stephens KU, Grew D, Chin K, et al. Excess mortality in the aftermath of Hurricane Katrina: a preliminary report. *Disaster Med Public Health Preparedness.* 2007;1:15–20.

3. Rodriguez J, Vos F, Below R, Guha-Sapir D. *Annual Disaster Statistical Review 2008: The Numbers and Trends.* Brussels, Belgium: Center for Research on the Epidemiology of Disasters; 2009. http://www.cred.be/sites/default/files/ADSR_2008.pdf. Accessed November 19, 2009.

4. Centers for Disease Control and Prevention. Natural disasters and severe weather. http://emergency.cdc.gov/disasters/. Accessed August 31, 2009.

5. Federal Emergency Management Agency. Disaster information. http://www.fema.gov/hazard/index.shtm. Accessed August, 31, 2009.

6. National Oceanic and Atmospheric Administration. NOAAWatch: NOAA's all hazard monitor. http://www.noaawatch.gov/. Accessed August 31, 2009.

7. National Weather Service, National Oceanic and Atmospheric Administration. *Summary of Natural Hazard Statistics for 2008 in the United States.* http://www.nws.noaa.gov/om/hazstats/sum08.pdf. Accessed August 31, 2009.

8. World Health Organization. *WHO Report on Infectious Diseases: Removing Obstacles to Healthy Development.* Geneva, Switzerland: WHO; 1999.

9. Centers for Disease Control and Prevention. Foodborne illness. http://www.cdc.gov/ncidod/dbmd/diseaseinfo/foodborneinfections_g.htm. Accessed August 31, 2009.

10. Centers for Disease Control and Prevention. Water-related diseases, contaminants, and injuries. http://www.cdc.gov/healthywater/disease/. Accessed August 31, 2009.

11. World Health Organization. Burden of disease and cost-effectiveness estimates. http://www.who.int/water_sanitation_health/diseases/burden/en/index.html. Accessed August 31, 2009.

12. Agency for Toxic Substances and Disease Registry. *Hazardous Substances Emergency Events Surveillance: Annual Report 2005.* Atlanta, GA: US Department of Health and Human Services; 2005. http://www.atsdr.cdc.gov/HS/HSEES/Annual2005.pdf. Accessed August 31, 2009.

13. US Fire Administration. Fire statistics: all structures. http://www.usfa.dhs.gov/statistics/national/all_structures.shtm. Accessed August 31, 2009.

14. National Highway Traffic Safety Administration. *Traffic Safety Facts, 2007 Data: Overview.* Publication DOT HS 810 993. Washington, DC: NHTSA National Center for Statistics and Analysis; 2008. http://www-nrd.nhtsa.dot.gov/Pubs/810993.PDF. Accessed August 31, 2009.

15. Arnold JL, Halpern P, Tsai M, Smithline, H. Mass casualty terrorist bombings: a comparison of outcomes by bombing type. *Ann Emerg Med.* 2004;43:263–273.

16. Pachauri RK, Reisinger A, eds. *Climate Change 2007: Synthesis Report. Contribution of Working Groups I, II, and III to the Fourth Assessment Report of the Intergovernmental Panel on Climate Change (IPCC).* Geneva, Switzerland: IPCC; 2008. Available at http://www.ipcc.ch/#. Accessed August 31, 2009.

17. Costello A, Abbas M, Allen A, Ball S, Bell S, Bellamy R, et al. Managing the health effects of climate change. *Lancet.* 2009; 373:1693–1733. Available at http://www.ucl.ac.uk/global-health/ucl-lancet-climate-change.pdf. Accessed August 31, 2009.

18. Karl TR, Melillo JM, Peterson TC, eds. *Global Climate Change Impacts in the United States: A State of Knowledge Report from the U.S. Global Change Research Program.* New York: Cambridge University Press; 2009. Available at http://www.globalchange.gov/usimpacts. Accessed August 31, 2009.

CHAPTER TWO

Personal Preparedness

2.1 PURPOSE

This chapter discusses the importance of personal preparedness for disasters and public health emergencies and the need for health professionals and others to become involved in local disaster planning and management efforts. The likelihood of experiencing some type of disaster affects everyone, and it is necessary to consider disaster preparedness in the context of personal health and safety.

2.2 LEARNING OBJECTIVES

After completing this chapter, readers should be able to:

➤ Demonstrate knowledge of the key components of, and the ability to prepare, a personal/family disaster plan.

➤ List potential hazards that need to be considered before entering the scene when given a disaster or public health emergency scenario.

➤ List by priority the immediate actions and precautions that are essential for preservation of personal and public safety according to the all-hazards approach to disaster management.

➤ Identify all appropriate authorities who should be contacted when given a disaster or public health emergency scenario.

➤ Identify informational resources for health professionals and the public regarding preparedness, response, and recovery in a disaster or public health emergency.

➤ Identify effective strategies to protect and ensure access to medical records and other valuable personal, family, and business documents in a disaster or public health emergency.

2.3 DISASTER MEDICINE AND PUBLIC HEALTH PREPAREDNESS COMPETENCIES ADDRESSED

This chapter addresses the following competencies as delineated in Appendix E of this manual.

➤ Explain key components of regional, community, institutional, and personal/family disaster plans.

➤ Describe immediate actions and precautions to protect yourself and others from harm in a disaster or public health emergency.

➤ Describe emergency communication and reporting systems and procedures for contacting family members, relatives, coworkers, and local authorities in a disaster or public health emergency.

➤ Describe informational resources that are available for health professionals and the public to prepare for, respond to, and recover from disasters and public health emergencies.

➤ Describe solutions for ensuring the continuity of supplies and services to meet the medical and mental health needs of yourself, your family, office practice, institution, and community in a disaster, under various contingency situations (eg, mass evacuation, mass sheltering, prolonged shelter-in-place).

2.4 OPENING VIGNETTE

During the past year, your town experienced exceptionally wet weather, causing near-record water levels in the river that runs through the heart of town. Following a heavy winter snowfall, the rains returned in early spring, adding more water to the already saturated soil. During the winter, a 20-inch layer of frost formed under much of the ground in the region and has not yet melted. Any rainwater that is seeping through the soil hits the frost barrier and runs off. There is just nowhere for the water to go. Three to four inches of rain is forecast over the next few days, which is expected to cause significant flooding. People along the river are being advised to prepare to evacuate their homes and businesses.

Would you be prepared to evacuate your home or business at a moment's notice? Where would you go? What personal items would you take with you? Do you have adequate insurance to cover any losses? Would you be able to report to, and function effectively at, your critical job?

2.5 PERSONAL AND FAMILY PLANNING[1,2]

Disasters can strike quickly and without warning, forcing community residents to evacuate their neighborhoods or stay at home for days. In a mass casualty event, individuals and communities will likely have to deal with an increased demand for medical resources, especially in rural areas and when local emergency medical services and hospitals are overwhelmed. The first minutes or hours are the most critical for seriously injured persons. During this time, health professionals and other skilled emergency responders will probably not be available at the disaster scene. Even when they arrive, emergency responders and relief workers cannot reach all affected people right away.

Everyone should think about what to do in a disaster, particularly if water, gas, electricity, or telephones are cut off for a long period of time. In such situations, local citizens can help give immediate assistance at a time when rapid intervention may be essential for survival. Until help arrives, citizens will be the "first responders" to care for injured victims. To prepare for such situations, all citizens should be able to:

➤ Recognize and protect themselves from potential dangers and hazards

➤ Know how and when to call for help

➤ Be willing and able to help without interfering with organized response efforts

➤ Know how to provide critical life support

Medical emergencies and disasters can occur at any time and in any place, and frequently require the assistance of skilled bystanders. Most injuries can be prevented by developing the situational awareness to recognize potential danger and take appropriate safety precautions. In serious life-threatening emergencies, knowledge of critical skills such as how to perform cardiopulmonary resuscitation (CPR) and how to control excessive bleeding can save lives.

2.5.1   Elements of a Personal/Family Disaster Plan

The best way to make homes and communities safer is to be prepared before disaster strikes. This can be done through thoughtful planning and can ensure that when a disaster occurs, people can respond safely and effectively. Personal and family planning and preparation enable community preparation. In this course readers will learn the elements that make up the recognition of, response to, management of, and recovery from an event and its consequences by using the DISASTER Paradigm™ (D, detect; I, incident management; S, security and safety; A, assess hazards; S, support; T, triage and treatment; E, evacuation; R, recovery). Just as important is the preparedness that is critical for effective disaster response. A useful acronym is PRE-DISASTER: P for planning and practice, R for resilience, and E for education and training. It is important for all family members to know how to react in a disaster or other emergency. Families should talk about disasters that are likely to happen in their area and how to prepare for each type. The family disaster plan should be practiced at least twice each year so that everyone will remember how to react in an emergency. In any disaster, the best protection is knowing what to do.

Typical questions addressed by a family disaster plan are how to take care of oneself and loved ones, where to go, and how to meet and communicate with others. Backup plans should be made for children in case the parents are unable to get home in an emergency. Children should know or have contact information with them. Family planning and preparedness can assist those who have a critical role to play in responding to a disaster in their community.

Sharing plans and communicating in advance is a good strategy. This includes talking to neighbors about how families can work together. Someone may have special equipment, like a portable generator, or expertise such as medical knowledge that might help in a crisis. Someone should be designated to check on elderly or disabled neighbors.

Emergency plans also should be standard in the workplace. Most often, these are created and then forgotten. Employees should ask the following questions about their workplace response plans:

➤ Is there one?

➤ Where is it located?

➤ What does it contain?

➤ What are each employee's specific responsibilities?

Similar questions should be asked about emergency plans for local schools, day care centers, and elder care centers. Individuals should take the time to research these plans before they need to be implemented.

A family disaster plan is simple to create. The process begins with gathering family members and making sure that each person is well informed about potential hazards and community action plans. Discussion should include what to do if family members are not home when an emergency alert or other warning is given. In addition, the following topics should be discussed:

➤ *Emergency alert systems.* All community members should know their local warning system. In the event of a disaster, local radio and television stations will provide information on evacuation routes, temporary shelters, and other emergency procedures. Depending on the circumstances, any one of three protective actions (shelter-in-place, prepare to evacuate, or evacuate) may be appropriate. In emergencies, the news media will be relied on to communicate essential messages to the public. It is important to have the means (eg, a battery-powered radio) to get up-to-date information and instructions.

➤ *Escape routes.* Families should talk about and decide on escape routes in the home for all family members. Each individual should know the fastest way out of the home and how not to become trapped.

➤ *Places to meet.* A place should be designated for family members to meet if an emergency happens. A meeting place away from home (a neighbor or relative's house or even a street corner) should be agreed on for family members to get together if they were separated in an emergency.

➤ *Emergency contacts.* Each family member should have an emergency list with the name, address, and telephone number of the meeting place. Children who are old enough should be helped to memorize this information.

➤ *Evacuation routes.* Many types of emergencies (eg, fire, flood, earthquake, hurricane) may lead to evacuation. The amount of time available to leave the area will depend on the type of disaster. If the event is weather related, such as a hurricane that can be monitored, there might be a day or two to get ready. Other disasters allow no time for family members to gather even the most basic necessities. In such situations, it is essential to plan ahead.

➤ *Family communications.* Families may not be together when a disaster strikes, so it is important to plan in advance on how members will contact each other in different situations. Emergency telephone numbers should be kept where family members can find them. It is a good idea to designate a family contact, out of the affected area, with whom family members can check in if separated during an emergency or if the family's home is damaged or family members cannot return safely.

➤ *Utility shutoff and safety.* In the event of a disaster, it may be necessary to shut off the utility service (water, electricity, natural gas) at home. Residents should learn the location of utility shutoff valves and circuit breakers and how to turn them off.

➤ *Local shelters.* Emergency plans should never rely on a single shelter. Community members should know the locations of all potential shelters that are available for their community. Shelters are often located in public school buildings; information on locations is available from the local Office of Emergency Management Web site or local government Web site.

➤ *School emergency plans.* It is helpful to find out what local school districts and day care centers plan to do in the event of an emergency. Many districts stagger hours so that schools can share buses, and therefore they may not be able to evacuate all the schools at the same time. Children should be taught where to meet parents in the event that schools are evacuated or an early release occurs.

➤ *Insurance and important documents.* Arrangements should be made to back up or otherwise secure important records, documents, and files.

➤ *Care for pets.* It is advisable to avoid leaving pets behind. Pets most likely cannot survive on their own, and if they do, their owners may not be able to find them when they return. Because pets are not allowed in many emergency shelters, pet owners should find out in advance whether the location to which they plan to evacuate will allow pets; if not, they should find out where they can shelter pets locally.

➤ *Care for livestock.* Livestock should be evacuated whenever possible. All animals should have some form of identification that will allow owners to identify them later. Arrangements for evacuation, including routes and places to take the animals, should be made in advance. If evacuation is not possible, a decision must be made whether to move large animals to available shelter or move them outside. This decision should be based on the type of disaster and the condition and location of the animal shelter.

➤ *First aid and safety skills.* It is important that family members know how to administer first aid and CPR and how to use an automated external defibrillator and a fire extinguisher. The American Red Cross, the National Safety Council, and other accredited providers offer first aid courses.

➤ *Staying informed.* More information is available from the agencies, organizations, Internet sites, and publications that are provided in this chapter as well as in Appendix F of this manual.

Selected Web-Based Personal Preparedness Resources

Personal preparedness resources can be found on the Internet sites of most state and local public health and emergency management agencies. The following national organizations also provide useful resources.

American Academy of Pediatrics (AAP)

The AAP "Children & Disasters" Web site (http://www.aap.org/disasters) provides information and resources for physicians, families, child care centers, schools, and policymakers on disaster preparedness and response issues affecting children.

American Red Cross

The American Red Cross Web site (http://www.redcross.org) and offices nationwide have excellent resources for answering questions and walking residents through appropriate disaster preparation steps. Many of their materials are available in multiple languages.

Centers for Disease Control and Prevention (CDC)

The CDC Web site (http://www.cdc.gov) is a comprehensive and authoritative resource on clinical and public health issues for health professionals and citizens worldwide. It is updated frequently to provide reliable information quickly. Developed with the American Red Cross, the CDC "Emergency Preparedness and You" Web site (http://emergency.cdc.gov/preparedness/) provides personal and family preparedness information.

Department of Homeland Security (DHS)

The Department of Homeland Security's Ready.gov campaign (http://www.ready.gov/) takes an all-hazards approach to preparedness and in many ways complements resources from the CDC and the American Red Cross. It is a good public resource that addresses basic planning and technical information for individuals, families, and businesses.

2.5.2 Components of a Disaster Supply Kit

After a disaster, individuals may be on their own for hours or days before out-side help is available. There also may be times, such as during a flood or a heavy winter storm, when residents are unable to leave their home for days. In other situations, they may be asked to leave at a moment's notice with very little time to pack personal belongings.

A *disaster supply kit* is a collection of basic items that family members may need in a disaster. Every household should have adequate food, water, and other supplies to last for at least 3 days and, if possible, for up to 2 weeks. The items that family members would most likely need while away from home should be kept in an easy-to-carry container (possible containers include a large, covered trash can; camping backpack; large suitcase; or duffle bag). Basic items that should be considered in a family disaster kit include:

➤ *Water*. Families should store at least a 3-day supply of water, allowing at least 1 gallon of water per person (and pets) per day.

➤ *Food*. The supply should include at least 3 days' worth of food that does not need refrigeration, preparation, or cooking and that requires little or no water. Food items that are compact and lightweight should be selected. Foods that will create thirst should be avoided. Good choices are salt-free items, whole-grain cereals, and canned foods with high liquid content. A 3-day supply of food for pets should be included, preferably in bags, not cans.

➤ *Clothing and bedding*. This should include at least one complete change of clothing and shoes per person. Sleeping bags or blankets should be pro-vided to keep warm.

➤ *Sanitation supplies*. These include toilet paper; soap; liquid detergent; feminine hygiene products (such as tampons and sanitary pads); personal hygiene items (such as hand sanitizer, deodorant, toothpaste, toothbrushes, combs, and brushes); lip balm; sunscreen; plastic garbage bags and ties (for personal sanitation uses); a plastic bucket with a tight lid; disinfectant; and household chlorine bleach.

➤ *Other supplies and equipment*. Additional items that are just as important, and that may prove to be critical, are listed in the Appendix at the end of this chapter.

2.5.3 Protection of Personal Assets

To determine whether individual properties or businesses are at risk in a disas-ter, local building officials, city engineers, or planning and zoning administrators should be consulted. They can tell whether the building is in a disaster-prone area and can usually provide information on how individuals can protect themselves, their houses, businesses, and properties from various hazards. In addition to seeking such guidance, the following measures are recommended.

➤ *Buying insurance.* Existing policies should be reviewed for the amount and extent of coverage to be sure it is adequate for all possible hazards. Property, health, and life insurance should be obtained for those who do not have them. People who live in a flood-prone area should consider purchasing flood insurance to reduce their risk of flood loss. Buying flood insurance to cover the value of a building and its contents will not only provide greater peace of mind but also speed the recovery if a flood occurs.

➤ *Inventorying home possessions.* Residents should make a record of personal property for insurance purposes. This should include photos or a video of the interior and exterior of the home. Personal belongings should be included in the inventory. Having an inventory of one's home provides security in ensuring that, no matter what happens (home invasion, natural disaster, or home tragedy), the necessary information will be available to insurance companies and other authorities to get one's life back on track.

➤ *Protecting important documents.* Important documents such as insurance policies, deeds, property records, and other papers should be stored in a safe place, such as a safe-deposit box, away from home. Copies of important documents should be included in the disaster supply kit. Without proof of who they are, what they own, and what coverage they have, people will find that getting assistance and rebuilding their lives after a disaster emergency is difficult and emotionally taxing. It is helpful to learn how to distinguish between replaceable and nonreplaceable documents and to choose an alternate storage location or backup system for these documents. A good resource is the "Emergency Financial First Aid Kit," a detailed listing of a range of critical documents, available from Operation Hope (http://www.operationhope.org/smdev/lf1.php?id=187).

➤ *Stowing away some money.* Saving money in an emergency savings account that could be used in a crisis is worth considering. It is a good idea to keep a small amount of cash or traveler's checks at home in a safe and quickly accessible place.

2.6 PREVENTION, PREPAREDNESS, AND RESILIENCE

Since September 11, 2001, most people have come to appreciate that the scope of disasters extends beyond natural disasters and environmental crises. Disasters can result from biologic, chemical, and radiologic terrorism, suicide bombings, and mass violence. They also can vary in magnitude, from large-scale events, requiring community evacuation, to small-scale emergencies, impacting the health and safety of individual citizens and their families. Now more than ever, communities need to be able to prepare for and respond quickly to critical incidents. All responders need to be trained and educated to react appropriately to various emergency situations, as well as to appreciate the physical, social, and emotional needs and outcomes that may arise during such events.

Disaster response and recovery operations can be physically and emotionally challenging. Hours can be long, under difficult conditions. Burnout can come easily if careful attention is not given to pacing oneself, having sufficient time to relax, and minimizing stress. In addition to possessing specific knowledge and skills related to disaster management, emergency responders must possess the fitness to respond and ability to maintain that fitness once deployed.

Resilience to emergency situations is a function of individual prevention, preparedness, and wellness. Today, many people are overweight and chronically stressed. Increasingly, people have come to understand the significance of their health and well-being, as sleep and exercise feel like luxuries, and they experience lack of connection with family, neighbors, and community and a decline in trust. Chronic inactivity, addictive behaviors such as tobacco and alcohol use, and poor diet are important factors that contribute to poor health.

Compounding the insidious stresses of modern life, most people will eventually encounter special challenges that test them and put their health and support systems at risk. For some, it is the stress of care-giving, job loss, home foreclosure, family dissolution, diagnosis of a serious illness, or the death of a loved one. For others, it is living with a chronic illness—diabetes, cancer, an addiction, or a major mental health condition. Evidence has demonstrated that those with chronic diseases (both mental and physical), the elderly, pregnant women, and children are even more vulnerable in large-scale disasters such as Hurricane Katrina.[3-7]

Prevention, preparedness, and wellness strategies are essential to help individuals develop the strength, resilience, and coping skills to deal with health challenges. Much has been learned about the importance of protective factors as simple as immunizations, exercise, good nutrition, adequate rest, healthy human interactions, and support from peers. Patient and employee assistance and substance abuse intervention programs, access to peer and professional counseling, and social inclusion for all are key to enhancing health and well-being. Personal disaster planning and training also can help build resilience by empowering people to deal with serious health emergencies.

2.7 WHEN DISASTER STRIKES

In a disaster, first responders and affected individuals must act quickly to protect themselves as well as help trapped and injured persons. Under these conditions, personal health and safety must remain a primary concern. Responders risk injury and illness from various hazards, such as contaminated water, fire, damaged power lines, and gas leaks, as well as from nails, broken glass, and other sharp objects in damaged or destroyed buildings. All responders need to be aware of their surroundings with an eye for things that seem unusual or out of place and thus may indicate a potential problem. This is part of surveillance, whether for law enforcement or public health.

Those affected by a disaster should trust their intuition and experience; if something doesn't seem right, it probably isn't. It is important to stay calm, use common sense, be patient, and think before acting. Instructions from authorities via telephone or media broadcasts, or at the scene, should be followed. Appendix D of this manual contains a series of "Tip Sheets" to help individuals prepare for and cope with various disaster situations.

2.7.1   Activation of the Emergency Response System

When a health emergency occurs, whoever is present should immediately dial 911 or the local emergency medical dispatch number on any available telephone and not hang up until help arrives. This action will provide, in most circumstances, a person trained to assist as those on the scene await the arrival of appropriate emergency medical personnel and vehicles. Staying on the telephone provides a person to talk with as the caller continues managing the situation until help arrives. If the caller is unable to speak or must walk away from the telephone to help another person, he or she should not hang up the telephone, as it may provide the operator a means to find the location while the call is still connected.

If the emergency involves family members, it is important to have quick access to the names and telephone numbers of physicians and other health personnel who provide regular care to the family. A list also should be maintained with contact information (complete names, addresses, and telephone numbers) of family members, legal guardians, and others who have responsibility for making health care decisions in an emergency. It is helpful to fill out the "Emergency Notification Form" in Appendix B of this manual.

If at least three attempts to access help by calling 911 or the local emergency medical dispatch number are unsuccessful for any reason, the next option is to call a local hospital, ambulance service, or police or fire department. The poison control center for the local area can also be contacted if a poisoning, ingestion of an unknown substance, or possible chemical exposure is suspected.

Paramedics and other ambulance personnel are usually available through various community resources

In Case of Emergency (ICE)

A recent practice that has gained widespread recognition is for individuals to make an entry in their cell telephone directory labeled "ICE" (for "In Case of Emergency") with the contact information for the person who should be called if they are ill or injured and cannot tell someone whom to call. Emergency medical and hospital personnel are now being taught to look for this information in cell telephone directories. In addition, if there is a "note filed" capability in the cell telephone, it can be used for key medical information in the ICE listing such as allergies, medications, and medical conditions.

Reporting Emergencies

In any disaster, early detection, rapid reporting, and immediate action are important to reduce casualties. Any suspected or confirmed emergency situation should be reported immediately by calling 911 or other local emergency medical dispatch number. Additional reporting requirements for first responders are listed in their standard operating procedures and local emergency response plans.

People who are sick or injured should first try to contact their physician to determine whether emergency medical care is warranted. If the physician is not available, 911 or other local emergency medical dispatch number should be called.

The Regional Poison Control Centers, contacted by calling 800-222-1222, can provide help in dealing with health effects from chemical poisoning and exposure.

such as the fire department, police department, and volunteer associations. Residents should learn about the emergency medical services that are available in their community before an emergency occurs. Paramedics should not be called for minor illnesses or injuries such as sprained ankles, minor cuts, or colds; they need to be available to treat people who have more serious conditions. Often people with minor injuries can be driven to the hospital by a family member or friend. A person who is taking someone to the hospital should call the ill or injured person's physician, if there is time, so that the physician can call the emergency department. This enables the staff to know what to expect, to prepare for the person's arrival, and to discuss the case with the physician.

2.7.2 Activation of the Public Health System

Typically, state regulations specify not only diseases or conditions that are reportable, but also who is responsible for reporting them, what information is required, how to report and to whom, and how quickly the information is to be reported. State regulations also may specify control measures to be implemented when a certain disease occurs.

How to Report.   Activation of the public health system requires notification of the most local component of the system. For hospital personnel, this may involve notification of the infection control nurse, hospital epidemiologist, or safety officer. For others, the most likely entry point into the public health system is the local health department. The local health department will notify the state health department, which will notify appropriate federal authorities if needed.

What to Report.   States develop legal reporting requirements using as a guide the list of communicable diseases recommended as part of the National Notifiable Disease Surveillance System (NNDSS), as well as state and local public health priorities.[8] The NNDSS list is developed and revised periodically by the CDC and the Council of State and Territorial Epidemiologists (CSTE). Case definitions for each disease or condition are established and revised periodically by the CSTE and CDC. While most case definitions require laboratory test results to confirm a surveillance report, they have provisions to enable providers to report clinical cases without or in advance of laboratory confirmation. Case reports are usually considered confidential and are not available for public review.[9]

Specific diseases, conditions, and patient information that must be reported to local and state health officials differ by state. In general, a disease is listed if it causes morbidity or death, has the potential to affect large numbers of people, and can be controlled or prevented with proper interventions. In addition to specific diseases or conditions that have been established as reportable within a given state, health department regulations commonly specify two additional circumstances that require reporting: (1) the occurrence of any outbreak or unusually high incidence of any disease; and (2) the occurrence of any unusual disease of public health importance.

When a report is made, it is important to include all available information that may be of value in the clinical decision-making process. At a minimum, this should include demographic information (eg, patient name, address, telephone number), clinical information, and any available laboratory information.

When to Report.   When to report is as important as what to report. State laws specify timeframes for reporting certain diseases and conditions to public health authorities once a diagnosis is confirmed. Some diseases are immediately report-able because they require a public health response. These include diseases caused by possible bioterrorism agents (eg, anthrax, pneumonic plague, smallpox, and tularemia) as well as cases of measles, bacterial meningitis, and pertussis, among others.

Prevention of a public health emergency rests on early detection, rapid report-ing, and immediate response. The call from an alert health professional who has observed an unusual disease, even if uncertain about the diagnosis, may provide valuable clues to public health authorities that could lead to the early detection of a bioterrorist event or emerging epidemic.

Early detection may expedite implementation of public health control mea-sures to save lives by minimizing the spread of a potentially highly contagious disease. So, when in doubt, health care professionals should contact the health department.

Public Health Agency Contact Information

Health professionals should notify local public health authorities to report specific diseases or conditions as required by the state, as well as to report the occurrence of any disease outbreak, an unusually high incidence of any disease, and the occurrence of any unusual disease of public health importance.

The following links can be used to locate local and state health agencies:

➤ For a directory of local/regional public health agencies: http://www.naccho.org/about/lhd/

➤ For a directory of state public health agencies: http://www.cdc.gov/mmwr/international/relres.html

The contact information may be recorded on the "Emergency Notification Form," which is provided in Appendix B of this manual.

2.7.3   Reporting of Terrorism-Related Events

In the fall of 2001, public health officials in a number of communities had to deal with claims that anthrax or other bioterrorism agents had been released in their vicinities. In responding to these threats, considerable variation existed in the procedures used by local public health officials, particularly for communicating and notifying other public health officials and security agencies during the early response stages. To alleviate confusion, the CDC developed a standard communications protocol for use by local public health officials during the initial response to apparent acts of terrorism[10]:

1. If a health professional and/or health official in a local or state health department is notified about, or otherwise becomes aware of, apparent incidents or threats of terrorism, he or she should contact the Federal Bureau of Investigation (FBI), local public safety and law enforcement partners, and the local public health department. It is critical that the FBI be notified, because it is the designated agency for managing the legal investigation associated with a response to terrorist-related incidents. Typically, the Department of Homeland Security would be notified by state or federal law enforcement authorities. Close coordination between local and state authorities will be necessary in the event of actual or threatened instances of terrorism.

2. It may be difficult to immediately confirm that a terrorist incident is responsible for the occurrence of illness in the community. This is especially true for many of the critical biological agents that occur naturally in the United States (eg, *Bacillus anthracis*, *Francisella tularensis*). For situations that suggest the possibility of terrorism (albeit unconfirmed),

Notification of Authorities for Acts of Terrorism

Any actual or perceived act of terrorism should be reported to the FBI or local law enforcement agency. The CDC requests that all incidents of apparent or threatened terrorism be reported to the CDC by state public health officials immediately after notification of the FBI and local law enforcement authorities. State health officials should call the 24-hour notification telephone number (770-488-7100) at the CDC Emergency Preparedness and Response Branch.

More reporting information is available from the CDC Emergency Preparedness and Response Web site at http://emergency.cdc.gov/emcontact/.

A listing of FBI field offices is available at http://www.fbi.gov/contact/fo/fo.htm#cities.

local public health officials will work closely with their counterparts in the state health department. All state health departments have identified a state official in charge of the response. This person should be available 24 hours a day, 7 days a week, through a telephone number or other means of electronic communication provided to all local health departments. In many states, the person designated is the state epidemiologist.

2.8 HEALTH AND SAFETY CONSIDERATIONS FOR DISASTER RESPONDERS

In any disaster, health care professionals and other personnel must recognize and appreciate the potential risks and disruptions that are part of response operations. Sleeping, eating, personal time, and recreation patterns will likely be erratic. Persons may experience stress related to protecting their own safety and well-being, as well as that of others. Additional stress may be related to the care of casualties, the management of mass fatalities, and the unique situational restrictions and limitations encountered at the disaster scene.

All responders have a responsibility to be prepared to perform their duties and also to assess whether they are healthy enough to respond effectively. They must decide whether they can function in less than optimal circumstances and environments. Response personnel who are under medical care for acute and chronic problems should discuss their conditions with a physician or other health professional in advance of any disaster deployment.

Damage caused by natural and human-caused disasters creates myriad health and safety risks for affected populations and emergency responders. Depending on the event, there may be a large number of serious casualties, which may require search, rescue, and support operations under potentially hazardous and stressful conditions. Without proper precautions, additional casualties may result from secondary hazards such as structural collapse, excessive heat, motor vehicle crashes, downed power lines, ruptured gas mains, release of hazardous materials by fires or explosions, and infectious disease outbreaks.

> **Protect Personal Safety**
>
> Any recognized or suspected hazard should be reported to appropriate authorities. Responders should not enter any disaster scene or take any action until authorities determine it is safe. Protecting themselves from becoming a casualty is the number 1 priority.

Before entering any disaster scene, it is important that responders protect themselves through the selection and use of appropriate personal protective equipment (PPE). The appropriate level of protection depends on the unique situation and is discussed in greater detail in the basic and advanced National Disaster Life Support™ (NDLS™) courses. The PPE is intended to minimize contact with contaminated persons, objects, and environments. It protects those body parts that are vulnerable to exposure and penetration: the skin, the mouth, the eyes, the nose, and the respiratory tract.

Types of PPE are classified as either "simple" or "advanced." The simple level of protection includes gloves, impermeable gowns, goggles, caps, and leg and shoe covers. This level of protection is common in health care facilities. Simple protection is suitable for most Core Disaster Life Support® providers and other persons without specialized PPE training and fit-testing. The advanced level of PPE includes supplied air, either self-contained or provided by an air hose, as well as whole-body protection by a chemical-resistant suit. This level of PPE should be reserved for trained personnel. In all cases, optimal scene safety requires selection of the proper equipment to be worn by the appropriate personnel in the correct setting.

Determination of the appropriate level of PPE to be used at the scene will be made by local response experts, such as hazardous materials (HAZMAT) personnel. Important considerations include the following:

➤ Is there an immediate danger to life or health?

➤ What agent was released?

➤ How was the agent released (eg, gas, liquid, particles)

➤ Is the release site confined?

➤ How close by is the release site?

➤ What is each responder's expected role and job duty during the event?

The actions of a first responder at a HAZMAT event, as found in Guide 111 of the Emergency Response Guidebook, are as follows:[11]

➤ Stay upwind

➤ Stay out of low-lying areas

➤ Keep unnecessary people away

➤ Isolate 300 feet (100 meters) in all directions

When it is deemed safe for people to return to their homes after a disaster, they also should take adequate precautions and follow the guidance of the local public health and public safety officials. Depending on the nature of the disaster, these may include wearing boots and work gloves, and being sure to cover all exposed areas of the body. If possible, watertight boots with a steel toe and insole, gloves, protective clothing (long pants, long-sleeved shirts), and safety glasses should be worn during cleanup operations; sandals and sneakers should not be worn because they will not prevent punctures, bites, or crush injuries. A hard hat should be worn if there is any danger of falling debris.

PPE Limitations

All forms of PPE have limitations:

➤ Proper use of advanced PPE requires specific training and fit-testing. Inexperienced persons donning advanced PPE cannot expect proper protection.

➤ No single type of PPE protects against all potential hazards.

➤ The PPE can itself create hazards (due to lack of heat dissipation, decreased vision, decreased mobility, decreased manual dexterity, and communications difficulties).

➤ Users cannot eat, drink, or use restroom facilities while wearing advanced PPE.

➤ Users must take precautions to prevent hyperthermia and dehydration.

More information about the uses and limitations of PPE is available on the website of the Occupational Safety and Health Administration (OSHA) at http://www.osha.gov/ SLTC/personalprotectiveequipment/index.html.

For more information on respirators and respirator safety, visit the National Institute for Occupational Safety and Health Web site at http://www.cdc.gov/niosh/npptl/.

Structural Instability. Water can weaken the walls and foundations of buildings. Pressure from water in the ground surrounding foundations can cause structural damage or collapse. The following are signs of unsafe structural conditions:

➤ Washed-out soil around the foundation

➤ Large cracks or gaps in the foundation

➤ Sagging roofs or ceilings

➤ Floors that bounce or give when walked on

➤ Doors or windows that appear out of alignment

While it may be necessary to remove standing water from the scene, no more than a third of the water should be pumped out each day to allow the building to settle gradually, avoiding further damage. No one should enter a building that may have structural damage until a qualified individual inspects it and determines that it is safe.

Electrical and Gas Hazards. Before entering a damaged building, responders should turn off the gas and electricity to avoid electrocution, fire, and explosions. They should be aware of flooded electrical circuits, downed power lines, broken or leaking gas lines, submerged furnaces or appliances, and flammable materials. To protect against fire-related injuries, the following steps should be taken:

➤ If the smell of gas is evident or a gas leak is suspected, the building should be immediately evacuated and the fire department or gas company called to check for leaks. The building should be reentered only after the leak is controlled and the area well ventilated.

➤ Availability of an adequate number of fire extinguishers and smoke detectors should be ensured and fire evacuation routes well marked.

➤ All fire exits should be confirmed to be clear.

➤ Only battery-powered flashlights should be used when a building is inspected. An open flame should never be used in a damaged area.

To help protect against electrical hazards:

➤ Awareness of overhead and underground power lines is necessary when debris is being cleared. Extreme caution is necessary when ladders and other equipment are moved near overhead power lines to avoid inadvertent contact.

➤ Care should be taken not to touch downed power lines or any object or water that is in contact with such lines. It is safest to treat all power lines as energized until it is confirmed that the lines have been deenergized.

➤ Responders should not touch electrical equipment if the ground is wet unless the power is off. If damage to an electrical system is suspected (for example, if the wiring has been under water, the smell of burning insulation is evident, wires are visibly frayed, or sparks are visible), the electrical system in the building should be turned off before work is begun. The power should not be turned back on until electrical equipment has been inspected by a qualified electrician.

➤ Deenergized power lines may become energized by a secondary power source such as a portable backup generator. When a generator is used, the main circuit breaker should be off before the generator is started. This will prevent inadvertent energization of power lines from backfeed electrical energy from generators and help protect utility line workers from possible electrocution.

➤ Any electrical equipment, including extension cords used in wet environments, must be marked as appropriate for use in wet locations and must be undamaged. All connections must be out of water. All cord-connected, electrically operated tools and equipment must be grounded or be double insulated.

➤ Ground-fault circuit interrupters (GFCIs) must be used in all wet locations. Portable GFCIs can be purchased at hardware stores and must be installed by a competent electrician.

Physical Dangers.   Responders should use caution when entering a disaster scene. Dangers may include sharp objects such as nails, broken glass, or metal fragments that can be hidden in water or mud, as well as slippery floors and surfaces. Materials or furniture in flooded areas may have absorbed water. They could weigh many times their normal weight. When moving heavy or wet objects, workers should:

➤ Use caution and always lift with their legs.

➤ Avoid back injuries by using teams of two or more people.

➤ Avoid lifting objects that weigh more than 50 pounds per person.

Carbon Monoxide.   Disaster cleanup may include the use of gas or diesel-powered pumps, generators, and tools. This equipment should never be used indoors or in confined spaces. These tools often give off carbon monoxide, a colorless, odorless gas. When such equipment is used outdoors, it should be ensured that exhaust does not enter buildings. Carbon monoxide poisoning may lead to sickness or death. Urgent medical attention is required if the following symptoms occur:

➤ Dizziness

➤ Headaches

➤ Nausea

➤ Excessive tiredness

➤ Cherry-red skin color—a late and critical sign

Chemicals and Contaminants. Workers should use extreme caution when handling containers with unknown substances or known toxic substances (for example, floating containers of household or industrial chemicals). Most homes and businesses store potentially hazardous chemicals that can be released in a disaster. This includes cleaning chemicals, gasoline, paints, solvents, and pesticides. Floodwater can dislodge containers that hold these chemicals. If working in an area that may be contaminated, workers should:

➤ Wear protective clothing and respirators to avoid skin contact or inhalation of vapors.

➤ Contain the spill area if possible.

➤ Construct a dam to prevent chemicals from spreading.

➤ Put smaller containers that are leaking into larger containers.

Some symptoms of pesticide poisoning include:

➤ Headache

➤ Nausea

➤ Diarrhea

➤ Sweating

➤ Breathing difficulty

➤ Tremors or convulsions

These symptoms usually appear immediately or within a few hours after exposure.

Molds and Mildew. When temperatures exceed 70°F (21°C), mold growth can occur on many surfaces. Large numbers of mold spores can trigger allergic reactions, infections, and other respiratory problems, as well as poisoning. If a mold problem is detected, attempts should be made to isolate it by:

➤ Sealing off the area or objects that have mold growth

➤ Keeping air movement to a minimum

➤ Avoiding opening and closing doors

➤ Blocking ventilation systems so that spores cannot spread to other areas

To limit exposure to airborne mold, workers should consider wearing an N95 respirator, which is available at most hardware stores and from companies that advertise on the Internet (the cost is about $12 to $25, depending on quantity). Some N95 respirators resemble a paper dust mask with a nozzle on the front; others are made primarily of plastic or rubber and have removable cartridges that trap most of the mold spores to prevent them from entering. To be effective, the respirator or mask must fit properly, so it is important to carefully follow the instructions supplied with the respirator. Note that OSHA requires that respirators fit properly (fit testing) when used in occupational settings. More information is available from OSHA at 800-321-OSHA or http://www.osha.gov.

Asbestos.   Asbestos was commonly used for insulation, ceilings, and floorings in buildings until the 1970s. Asbestos fibers do not present a risk when they are enclosed. As asbestos-containing materials dry, however, asbestos fibers can flake off. If the fibers become airborne, they can be very dangerous. The fibers are microscopic and easily inhaled.

Lead.   Lead can present a hazard in flooded and otherwise damaged buildings. Many buildings constructed before 1978 were painted with materials containing high levels of lead. Lead from paint, chips, and dust can pose serious health hazards if not taken care of properly. Water can damage painted walls, causing the paint to crack and flake. Dust from the lead paint can be inhaled. Workers should take precautions to avoid exposure to lead dust when removing debris, or when remodeling or renovating after a disaster.

Wildlife.   After a disaster, animals can be forced out of their natural habitats and into unusual places. Snakes, insects, rodents, and other small animals can easily get into damaged structures. When surveying a disaster scene, workers should take the following precautions:

➤ Learn how to identify potentially harmful snakes, spiders, and insects in their area.

➤ Be aware of animals that carry rabies.

➤ Look for snakes, spiders, and animals around piles of debris or trash.

➤ Never expose hands or feet where animals may be hiding. Wear protective clothing, tall boots, and gloves.

➤ Use sticks or shovels to remove debris.

➤ If an animal is found, avoid sudden movement; if the workers remain still, the workers animal may leave. Workers should never corner an animal or try to catch it themselves but should call in a professional, such as an animal control officer.

2.9 DEALING WITH THE EMOTIONAL IMPACT OF DISASTERS[12-14]

In addition to the substantial impact that disasters can have on physical health, they place significant stress and psychological trauma on responders and affected populations. Experiencing a disaster can be one of the most difficult events a person can endure, and it can have both short- and long-term effects. Most people who experience a disaster, whether as a victim or as a responder, will have some type of psychological, physical, and/or emotional response to the event. This is normal. Common symptoms include the following:

➤ Fear

➤ Helplessness

➤ Worry

➤ Anger

➤ Confusion

➤ Difficulty concentrating

➤ Fatigue

➤ Tension

➤ Changes in sleep

➤ Loss of appetite

➤ Stress

It is possible to experience many of these symptoms at the same time. It is important to remember that most people who experience these symptoms will be able to return to normal functioning within a few weeks. Individuals may not be able to make sense out of what happened, which is normal.

There is no one way to feel after a tragic event, and people should not think that there is something wrong with them for feeling a certain way or if they respond differently than others. They may want to talk about the events that occurred and how they are feeling. This can be very helpful especially in a supportive environment. However, people should not feel as though they have to talk about the event if they do not want to.

Thinking Positively. It is helpful to think about one's abilities and capability to handle the situation. A positive outlook can increase a person's ability to perform under stressful situations and increase resistance to negative consequences.

Controlling Anxiety.   There are many ways in which people control their anxiety. Learning relaxation techniques such as deep breathing and progressive muscle relaxation can help control the negative physical and emotional response to anxiety.

Drugs or alcohol should not be used to aid in relaxing; these can have a rebound affect that increases anxiety. They may also impair judgment at a critical time when it is needed most.

Staying Informed.   After a disaster, it is important to obtain accurate information about what happened and what the community needs people to do to help or be safe. Newspapers, radio, and television are ways to get accurate local information. Getting accurate information from reliable sources will help residents know what actions and direction to take.

Staying Connected.   People bounce back from trauma when they feel connected and part of a team. They should reconnect with loved ones, neighbors, and coworkers. People may attend convocations and memorial services to heal as a community.

Seeking Help.   It should be remembered that feelings of fear, anger, anxiety, and depression following a traumatic event are natural. If these symptoms continue for several weeks after the event has passed, or if these feelings become overwhelming to the extent that a person cannot continue daily activities, he or she should consider talking to a physician or other mental health professional. Symptoms that may indicate a need for further evaluation include but are not limited to:

➤ Changes in eating and sleeping habits

➤ Prolonged physical problems such as stomach upset, back and neck aches, and headaches

➤ Inability to focus or concentrate on routine tasks or work

➤ Lack of interest in previously enjoyable activities

➤ Extreme fear of leaving one's home

➤ Prolonged irritability and significant mood swings

➤ Having flashbacks or nightmares or mentally replaying the events over and over

➤ Taking extreme measures to avoid the memories through the misuse of alcohol or other drugs

➤ Feeling hopeless, helpless, or that life is not worth living

➤ Feeling suicidal

➤ Having extreme anxiety such as panic attacks

2.10 EDUCATION AND TRAINING IN DISASTER MEDICINE AND PUBLIC HEALTH PREPAREDNESS

The need for trained responders is vital in the first minutes, hours, and even days after an event, when survivors may have no alternative to treating and caring for themselves, their families, coworkers, and neighbors. At times, survivors may be required to act independently for many hours after a disaster event until outside help arrives. To improve personal and community preparedness, all potential health system responders should seek disaster training to make sure they can:

➤ Recognize potential life-threatening situations and act appropriately, while protecting personal health and safety.

➤ Know how to contact and work with local emergency medical and public health systems.

➤ Make decisions with limited resources and limited information.

➤ Access reliable disaster health information and resources.

➤ Know about medical, social, and mental health resources that are available.

Everyone can benefit from learning basic first aid skills. Simple techniques such as clearing an airway or stopping heavy bleeding can make the difference between life and death. The more realistic the training, the more likely the trained person will be able to recall what to do in an emergency situation. The local American Red Cross chapter, the National Safety Council, or the local public health agency can provide information on first aid training courses in the area.

Health care professionals need ongoing training and education to ensure that they understand their particular roles, responsibilities, and contributions to the disaster health system. The coordinated and integrated response that communities and the nation as a whole must implement in a disaster makes it critical that public health, emergency medical services, and clinical personnel be trained in multidisciplinary settings. The NDLS Program addresses the important skills, competencies, and educational needs in disaster management and response that are common to multiple disciplines and professions. Curricula and training provide a consistent learning experience that includes (1) using an all-hazards approach; (2) covering the full spectrum of disaster mitigation, prevention, response, and recovery; (3) providing specific information to address clinical and public health aspects; mental health; ethical and legal issues; and the needs of particular at-risk populations (eg, children, pregnant women, the disabled,

Essential First Aid Skills for All Health System Responders
➤ Scene and casualty assessment
➤ Resuscitation
➤ Control of bleeding and treatment of shock
➤ Management of fractures and dislocations
➤ Care of the unconscious casualty
➤ Safe movement of injured persons

frail elderly); (4) using a common vocabulary (eg, glossary of terms and definitions) to provide standard information across professions; (5) providing a fundamental mutual understanding and working knowledge of the integrated roles and responsibilities of health professionals and other responders at a disaster scene; and (6) providing mechanisms to verify that learners have attained a defined level of knowledge and skill.

In 2008, a consensus-based educational framework and competency set was published from which educators could devise learning objectives and curricula in disaster medicine and public health preparedness, tailored to the needs of all health professionals.[15] The framework includes the delineation of core learning domains and competencies targeted at three broad health personnel categories (ie, informed worker/student, practitioner, and leader). A learning matrix was developed to allow health educators and accreditation entities to incorporate the competencies at any desired proficiency level. These competencies provide the basis for all NDLS training. They can be used to update and revise job descriptions, outline required training, and assess progress toward meeting preparedness goals. The complete set of competencies is provided in Appendix E of this manual.

2.11 VOLUNTEER OPPORTUNITIES

Health professionals and others should learn about opportunities that are available to become more involved in local disaster preparedness and response efforts. This includes opportunities to volunteer in local disaster relief. Information on many disaster relief agencies and opportunities is available on the Web site of the National Volunteer Organizations Active in a Disaster at http://www.nvoad.org.

The Citizen Corps (http://www.citizencorps.gov/) was created to help coordinate volunteer activities to make communities safer, stronger, and better prepared to respond to any emergency situation (eg, crime threats, terrorism, and disasters). The Citizen Corps is coordinated nationally by the Federal Emergency Management Agency (FEMA). In this capacity, FEMA works closely with other federal entities, state and local governments, first responders and emergency managers, the volunteer community, and the Corporation for National and Community Service. The five Citizen Corps programs are as follows:

➤ The *Community Emergency Response Team (CERT) Program* (http://www.citizencorps.gov/cert/index.shtm), administered by FEMA, prepares people to help themselves, their families, and their neighbors in the event of a disaster in their community. Through CERT, citizens can learn about disaster preparedness and receive training in basic disaster response skills such as fire safety, light search and rescue, and disaster medical operations. With this training, volunteers can provide immediate assistance to victims before first responders arrive on scene. CERT volunteers also participate in community preparedness outreach activities.

➤ The *Fire Corps* (http://www.firecorps.org) promotes the use of citizen volunteers to support and augment the capacity of resource-constrained fire and emergency service departments at all levels: volunteer, career, and combination (career/volunteer). Fire Corps is funded through the Department of Homeland Security and is managed and implemented through a partnership between the National Volunteer Fire Council and the International Association of Fire Chiefs.

➤ The *Medical Reserve Corps (MRC) Program* (http://www.medicalre servecorps.gov) reports directly to the US Surgeon General. The MRC aims to improve the health and safety of communities across the country by organizing and utilizing public health, medical, and other volunteers who donate their time and expertise to prepare for and respond to emergencies. Volunteer MRC units accomplish this mission by supplementing existing emergency and public health resources during local emergencies.

➤ *USAonWatch* (http://www.usaonwatch.org) is the face of the National Neighborhood Watch Program. The program is managed nationally by the National Sheriffs' Association in partnership with the US Department of Justice. USAonWatch empowers citizens to become active in homeland security efforts through community participation. This is accomplished through information, training, technical support, and resources to local law enforcement agencies and citizens.

➤ The *Volunteers in Police Service (VIPS) Program* (http://www.policevol unteers.org) serves as a gateway to information for law enforcement agencies and citizens interested in law enforcement volunteer programs. The program's ultimate goal is to enhance the capacity of state and local law enforcement agencies by incorporating the time and skills that volunteers can contribute to a community law enforcement agency. The International Association of Chiefs of Police manages the VIPS Program in partnership with the US Department of Justice.

It is important to realize that anyone, regardless of expertise or level of training, can participate in disaster preparedness activities in their community. Across the United States, community leaders and citizen volunteers are working on the development and refinement of local plans that will be used in the event of a local, regional, or national emergency. These hometown meetings serve as important opportunities to meet with state and national emergency response partners who will be working with communities in an emergency and to learn about their preparations and plans.

The more individuals know, the better able they will be to protect themselves and their communities in the event of a serious disaster or other public health emergency. The bottom line is to be prepared, stay informed, and get involved.

The National Disaster Medical System

The National Disaster Medical System (NDMS) is a federally coordinated response system that supplements state and local emergency resources during disasters or major emergencies, and provides support to the military and the Department of Veterans Affairs medical systems in caring for US casualties from overseas armed conflicts. The NDMS comprises individuals with expertise and experience in a wide range of professions, including the clinical, public health, forensics, and mortuary sciences. Response teams are positioned nationwide with personnel who have completed an application process and met prerequisite training requirements. Qualified individuals are assigned to designated teams, which receive additional training in disaster management and response. NDMS personnel are required to maintain appropriate and current professional certifications and licensure in their discipline. Opportunities to serve in the NDMS include:

➤ Disaster Medical Assistance Teams (DMATs) (this includes special teams for pediatrics, burns, search and rescue, and mental health)

➤ Disaster Mortuary Operational Response Teams

➤ National Pharmacy Response Teams

➤ National Veterinary Response Team

For more information, visit the NDMS website at http://www.hhs.gov/aspr/opeo/ndms/index.html.

2.12 SUMMARY

All citizens should be vigilant of their surroundings with an eye for things that seem unusual. They should be wary of circumstances that are out of place and thus may indicate a potential problem. This is part of surveillance, whether for law enforcement or public health. Citizens should stay calm, use common sense, be patient, and think before they act. They should follow instructions from authorities via telephone or media broadcasts or at the scene.

Everyone should think about and plan for what to do in a disaster, particularly if basic services and utilities are cut off for a long period of time. Until help arrives, citizen bystanders will be the "first responders" to care for injured victims. In such situations, they need to be able to:

➤ Recognize potential life-threatening situations and act appropriately, while protecting personal health and safety.

➤ Know how to contact and work with local emergency medical and public health systems.

➤ Make decisions with limited resources and limited information.

➤ Access reliable disaster health information and resources.

➤ Know about medical, social, and mental health resources that are available.

Reporting Emergencies. In any disaster, early detection, rapid reporting, and immediate action are important to reduce casualties. Any suspicious or confirmed emergency situation should be reported immediately by calling 911 or other local emergency medical dispatch number. Additional reporting requirements for first responders are listed in their standard operating procedures and local emergency response plans. Any actual or perceived act of terrorism should be reported to the FBI or local law enforcement agency.

Health professionals should notify local public health authorities to report specific diseases or conditions as required by the state, as well as to report the occurrence of any disease outbreak, an unusually high incidence of any disease, and the occurrence of any unusual disease of public health importance.

Activating the Public Health System. Activation of the public health system typically occurs at the local level. Activation of this system needs to occur as soon as possible during an evolving public health emergency, so that appropriate prevention and control measures can be implemented to limit disease spread. Health professionals should be on constant alert for unusual disease occurrences and patterns and report them to public health authorities.

2.13 SELF-LEARNING SCENARIOS

After completing the CDLS® course and each of the chapters in this manual, take time to work through the 4 scenarios presented in Appendix A. The scenarios are designed for the application and reinforcement of "core" concepts and principles in disaster life support.

REFERENCES

1. Subbarao I, Lyznicki J, James JJ, eds. *American Medical Association Handbook of First Aid and Emergency Care.* New York, NY: Random House; 2009.

2. Federal Emergency Management Agency. *Are You Ready? An In-Depth Guide to Citizen Preparedness.* Washington, DC: FEMA; 2004. http://www.fema.gov/areyouready/. Accessed August 24, 2009.

3. Aldrich N, Benson WF. Disaster preparedness and the chronic disease needs of vulnerable older adults. *Prev Chronic Dis* [serial online]. 2006;3:1–7. http://www.cdc.gov/pcd/issues/2008/jan/07_0135.htm. Accessed November 13, 2009.

4. Sharma AJ, Weiss EC, Young SL, et al. Chronic disease and related conditions at emergency treatment facilities in the New Orleans area after Hurricane Katrina. *Disaster Med Public Health Preparedness*. 2008;2:27–32.

5. Brodie M, Weltzien E, Altman D, Blendon RJ, Benson JM. Experiences of Hurricane Katrina evacuees in Houston shelters: implications for future planning. *Am J Public Health*. 2006;96:1402–1408.

6. The Hurricane Katrina Community Advisory Group, Kessler RC. Hurricane Katrina's impact on the care of survivors with chronic medical conditions. *J Gen Intern Med*. 2007;22:1225–1230.

7. Rath B, Donato J, Duggan A, et al. Adverse health outcomes after Hurricane Katrina among children and adolescents with chronic conditions. *J Health Care Poor Underserved*. 2007;18:405–417.

8. Centers for Disease Control and Prevention. *Nationally Notifiable Infectious Diseases*. http://www.cdc.gov/ncphi/disss/nndss/phs/infdis.htm. Accessed August 24, 2009.

9. Centers for Disease Control and Prevention. Case definitions for infectious conditions under public health surveillance. *MMWR*. 1997;46(No. RR-10). http://www.cdc.gov/epo/dphsi/casedef/index.htm. Accessed August 24, 2009.

10. Centers for Disease Control and Prevention. *Protocols: Interim Recommended Notification for Local and State Public Health Department Leaders on the Event of a Bioterrorist Incident*. http://www.bt.cdc.gov/EmContact/Protocols.asp. Accessed August 24, 2009.

11. Transport Canada. *Emergency Response Guidebook 2008*. http://www.apps.tc.gc.ca/saf-sec-sur/3/erg-gmu/erg/ergmenu.aspx. Accessed January 6, 2009.

12. Centers for Disease Control and Prevention. *Coping With a Disaster or Traumatic Event*. http://www.bt.cdc.gov/mentalhealth/. Accessed August 24, 2009.

13. Federal Emergency Management Agency. *Coping With Disaster*. http://www.fema.gov/rebuild/recover/cope.shtm. Accessed August 24, 2009.

14. Substance Abuse and Mental Health Services Administration, National Mental Health Information Center. Hurricane and other disaster relief information: publications on mental health & disaster issues. http://mentalhealth.samhsa.gov/cmhs/Katrina/pubs.asp. Accessed August 24, 2009.

15. Subbarao I, Lyznicki JM, Hsu EB, et al. A consensus-based educational framework and competency set for the discipline of disaster medicine and public health preparedness. *Disaster Med Public Health Preparedness*. 2008;2:57–68.

APPENDIX

Disaster Supplies Checklist

➤ Water. Have at least a 3-day supply of water and store at least 1 gallon of water per person per day.

➤ Food. Store at least a 3-day supply of food that doesn't need refrigeration, preparation, or cooking and requires little or no water. Select food items that are compact and lightweight. Avoid foods that will make you thirsty. Choose salt-free items, whole grain cereals, and canned foods with high liquid content.

➤ Clothing and bedding. Include at least one complete change of clothing and shoes per person. Provide sleeping bags or blankets to keep warm.

➤ Sanitation supplies. Include toilet paper; soap; liquid detergent; feminine hygiene products (such as tampons and sanitary pads); personal hygiene items (such as deodorant, toothpaste, toothbrushes, comb and brush); lip balm; sunscreen; plastic garbage bags and ties (for personal sanitation uses); a plastic bucket with tight lid; disinfectant; and household chlorine bleach.

➤ First aid kit

➤ Portable, battery-operated radio and extra batteries; preferably this should be a National Oceanic and Atmospheric Administration (NOAA) all-hazard alert radio. The NOAA station will include instructions on whether residents should stay in their homes, when to evacuate, and the status of the emergency event. Such radios can be purchased at a local electronics store.

➤ Flashlight and extra batteries

➤ Cash or traveler's checks, credit and ATM cards (although the latter may not work in a major disasters, possibly for days or weeks); it is recommended that $500 in cash be kept securely in the house and immediately accessible

➤ Extra set of house and car keys

➤ Manual can opener

➤ Fire extinguisher (small canister, ABC type)

➤ Small tent

➤ Mess kits, or paper cups and plates and plastic utensils

➤ Basic tools (such as hammer, utility knife, pliers, screwdrivers, shovel, wrench to turn off household utilities)

➤ Compass

> Matches in a waterproof container

> Aluminum foil

> Plastic storage containers

> Signal flares

> Needles, thread

> Medicine dropper (this can be used to sanitize water by using 16 drops of unscented liquid chlorine bleach to a gallon of water)

> Whistle

> Plastic sheeting and duct tape

> Regional maps

> Portable generator

Special Items for Infants

These should include the following:

> Formula

> Diapers

> Bottles

> Pacifiers

> Powdered milk

> Medications

Special Items for Other Family Members

People with special health needs (for example, children, the elderly, pregnant women, and diabetic or disabled persons) may need to:

> Have extra eyeglasses, contact lenses, and hearing-aid batteries.

> Have extra wheelchair batteries.

> Keep a list of the style and serial number of medical equipment.

> Know where to find family medical insurance cards. The emergency kit should include photocopies of the cards, or extra copies can be requested from the health care insurance provider.

> Have a list of health professionals, relatives, or friends who should be notified in an emergency.

➤ Include prescription and nonprescription medications. Diabetic individuals should have a 1-week supply of insulin. Everyone should carry a current list of prescription medications with them at all times (including why they are taking the medicine, the doses, and the physician's and pharmacist's contact information). Physicians can be consulted about ways to ensure that individuals have a large enough supply of prescription medications for an emergency.

Pets

The following should be included in the kit to be able to properly care for pets:

➤ Clothing to help small pets keep warm

➤ For cats, litter box and litter

➤ Leash or harness

➤ Collar with ID and rabies tags

➤ Crate or carrier

➤ Food and water

➤ Medications

➤ Vaccination records

➤ List of pet shelters

➤ List of veterinarians

In addition, it is useful to have a microchip placed in each pet in case of loss or emergency.

Important Family Documents

Copies of the following documents should be kept in a waterproof, portable container, with the originals secured in a remote safe-deposit box:

➤ Wills

➤ Insurance policies

➤ Contracts

➤ Deeds

➤ Stocks and bonds

➤ Passports

➤ Social Security cards

➤ Immunization and other health records

➤ Bank account numbers

➤ Birth, marriage, and death certificates

➤ Mortgage records

➤ Motor vehicle records

It is also a good idea to keep photocopies of credit and identification cards.

Important Telephone Numbers and Addresses

A list should be kept of contact information for physicians, pharmacists, special needs service providers, and caregivers, as well as contact and meeting place information for family members. Having a contact system in place is important for the immediate family, but also for the extended family members and friends who will be worried about the family during a situation such as an emergency evacuation. Take the time to complete the "Emergency Notification Form," which is provided in Appendix B of this manual. Be sure it is current and accessible to all family members.

CHAPTER THREE

Community Preparation and Planning

3.1 PURPOSE

This chapter describes the elements of community and health care facility disaster planning and the need for active participation of the public and private health sectors in this process.

3.2 LEARNING OBJECTIVES

After completing this chapter, and considering the all-hazards approach to disaster planning and mitigation, readers will be able to:

➤ Identify common hazards that need to be addressed in any disaster plan.

➤ Describe essential components of regional, community, and institutional disaster plans.

➤ Define the term *vulnerable population* as it is used in the context of a disaster or public health emergency.

➤ Identify individuals and populations at greater risk for development of adverse health effects in a disaster or public health emergency.

➤ Identify basic communication modalities that can be used effectively to contact family members, relatives, coworkers, and local authorities.

3.3 DISASTER MEDICINE AND PUBLIC HEALTH PREPAREDNESS COMPETENCIES ADDRESSED

This chapter addresses the following competencies as delineated in Appendix E of this manual.

➤ Explain key components of regional, community, institutional, and personal/ family disaster plans.

➤ Identify individuals (of all ages) and populations with special needs who may be more vulnerable to adverse health effects in a disaster or public health emergency.

➤ Describe emergency communication and reporting systems and procedures for contacting family members, relatives, coworkers, and local authorities in a disaster or public health emergency.

3.4 OPENING VIGNETTE

On a typically hot Monday morning in July, a 98-car freight train rumbles toward your town at 45 mph. The train, which has recently left a chemical processing district, carries tank cars containing several hazardous chemicals, among them propane and chlorine. Approximately 2 miles north of town, a mechanical failure in the axle of 1 car causes that car and the 30 cars immediately behind it to derail. The wreckage includes numerous propane tank cars, as well as 6 chlorine tank cars. Fire department and law enforcement personnel, as well as the local hazardous materials (HAZMAT) team, arrive within 10 minutes and implement an incident command system. Intermittent explosions rock the scene as propane tanks in the wreckage ignite. Residents in the affected and adjacent communities are beginning to call emergency management and health authorities for information and instructions to protect themselves and their families.

Would your community be prepared for such an event? Would your community and local health care system be prepared?

3.5 REGIONAL AND COMMUNITY DISASTER PLANNING[1-5]

Disasters and other catastrophic emergencies strike locally, and communities must bear the ultimate responsibility for planning for and mobilizing emergency and health care resources to ensure adequate surge capacity for disaster response. State and federal governments have greater resources than the local community, but they need time to assemble and transport resources to affected communities. While they may supplement local resources over time, communities should

FIGURE 3-1

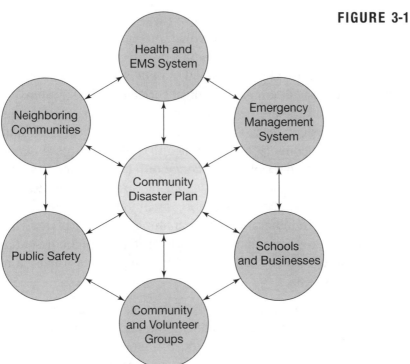

not plan on the state or federal government as either the initial or the primary resource in a mass casualty incident.

States and localities vary in size, population, risk, needs, and capabilities, which precludes development of "boilerplate" disaster preparedness and response plans. Plans must consider and accommodate regional and local needs, resources, and capabilities. Local businesses, schools, places of worship, and other community groups bring together individuals who know each other and who, because of their existing affiliations, are potentially ready to mobilize and work together. All of these groups need to be part of disaster planning and training. The more diverse the community, the greater the challenges, but with planning and cooperation a coordinated response will save lives and speed recovery (Figure 3-1).

To effectively prepare for and respond to an actual or threatened emergency, health officials and other emergency management personnel must collaborate with community partners to:

➤ Identify the types of events that might occur in their communities and regions

➤ Plan interagency emergency activities in advance to ensure a coordinated response to the consequences of credible threats

➤ Build the capabilities necessary to respond effectively to the consequence of those events

➤ Identify the type and nature of an event when it occurs

➤ Implement the planned response quickly and efficiently

➤ Mobilize resources to recover from the incident

Government agencies cannot achieve these objectives alone. Organized efforts to protect public health must involve all sectors of the community, including local public health agencies, hospitals, health care professionals, medical examiners, veterinarians, pharmaceutical suppliers, the media, emergency management agencies, the emergency medical services (EMS) system, local businesses, schools, law enforcement agencies, fire departments, and community organizations, as well as concerned citizens. In a disaster, local health authorities must prepare for the delivery of public health and health care services during the impact and postimpact phases. Agency officials will need to participate as full partners with the emergency management community in disaster response and recovery. To ensure such integration, they must participate in the development of and serve as an integral part of community disaster plans. They also must be present to ensure that community disaster plans include essentials for effective participation of public health and health care professionals in all training and response activities.

Planning efforts need to address education and training; identification and classification of resources, including personnel, supplies, and facilities; development of standard operating procedures, emergency response plans, and communications plans; and preplacement of essential supplies, countermeasures, and equipment in secure locations. Any large-scale emergency preparedness and response plan needs to consider the behavioral and emotional factors underlying human responses to trauma. Children are particularly at risk because they have not yet developed adult coping strategies and do not yet have the life experiences to help them understand what has happened.

Regional and community disaster plans must be developed and practiced well in advance of a serious event. Plans must be implemented through a continual cycle of preparation, training, equipping, exercising, evaluating, and taking corrective action to address gaps and deficiencies. Well-designed drills and exercises should be used to strengthen interagency relationships and to evaluate disaster plans, as well as to help emergency management and health authorities assess existing response capacities and capabilities and identify critical resourcing needs. All response agencies should be integrated into and participate with other response personnel during drills and exercises to better familiarize stakeholders with their respective roles and abilities. The time at which a disaster occurs is not the time for testing the plan.

3.6 FEDERAL PLANNING GUIDANCE

In 2007, the White House issued Homeland Security Presidential Directive-21 (HSPD-21) to establish a National Strategy for Public Health and Medical Preparedness.[6] This strategy builds on principles set out in Biodefense for the

21st Century (April 2004)[7] and the Homeland Security Presidential Directives described in this section. Four critical components of public health and medical preparedness were articulated as having the greatest potential to mitigate illness and death and thus to receive the highest priority in public health and medical preparedness efforts: biosurveillance, countermeasure distribution, mass casualty care, and community resilience. Implementation and realization of these efforts result from robust planning and guidance using the directives that are described below.

All government agencies must develop disaster response plans in accordance with the National Response Framework and the National Preparedness Guidelines to ensure that the public sector response integrates effectively with that of other stakeholders.[8, 9]

In 2003, President Bush issued Homeland Security Presidential Directive 5 (HSPD-5), which directed the Department of Homeland Security to develop and administer a National Incident Management System (NIMS).[10] As described in Chapter 4 of this manual, NIMS is a comprehensive, national approach to incident management that is applicable at all jurisdictional levels and across functional disciplines.[11] It provides a consistent nationwide framework to enable all government, private sector, and nongovernmental organizations to work together during domestic incidents.

HSPD-5 requires federal departments and agencies to make adoption of NIMS standards by state and local organizations a condition for federal preparedness assistance (grants, contracts, and other activities). To comply with HSPD-5, agencies and organizations at all levels are urged to follow NIMS standards and undertake measures to:

➤ Establish and coordinate emergency plans and protocols

➤ Integrate and coordinate activities and jurisdictions within their purview

➤ Establish guidelines and protocols to promote interoperability among jurisdictions and agencies

➤ Adopt guidelines and protocols for resource management

➤ Establish priorities for resources and other response requirements

➤ Establish and maintain multiagency command, control, and coordination mechanisms (Incident Command)

According to NIMS, jurisdictional plans must include:

➤ *Emergency operations plans*, which describe how the jurisdiction will respond to emergencies

➤ *Procedures*, which may include overviews, standard operating procedures, field operations guides, job aids, or other critical information needed for a response

➤ *Preparedness plans*, which describe how training needs will be identified and met, how resources will be obtained through mutual aid agreements, and the equipment required for the hazards faced by the jurisdiction

➤ *Corrective action and mitigation plans*, which include activities required to implement procedures based on lessons learned from actual incidents or training and exercises

➤ *Recovery plans*, which describe the actions to be taken to facilitate long-term recovery

The expanding challenge of preventing and preparing for major emergencies, whether natural or caused by human systems failure or conflict, has imposed the concept of "all-hazards" planning on governments at all levels.[5] In 2003, another presidential directive, HSPD-8, set forth all-hazards planning as the means to prepare governments to respond to a wide range of unpredictable threats and dangers.[12] Government agencies and organizations were instructed to develop plans that were adaptable and incorporated all potential hazards to reduce confusion during a disaster by using a consistent set of core responses. All-hazards planning saves time and effort by eliminating the need to develop multiple, redundant, and overly specific disaster plans.

The National Preparedness Guidelines define the capabilities that must be in place to prevent and respond to current and future threats, and they established measurable targets and priorities to guide national planning. Under these guidelines, state and local jurisdictions are encouraged to incorporate the following capabilities-based planning resources:

➤ The *National Planning Scenarios* give parameters for 15 terrorist attacks and natural disasters and provide the basis to define prevention, protection, response, and recovery tasks, as well as the capabilities required to perform them.

➤ The *Universal Task List* provides a comprehensive menu of some 1600 tasks to be performed by different disciplines at all levels of government to address disasters and other public health emergencies (such as those represented by the National Planning Scenarios). Although no single entity will perform every task, the list presents a common language and vocabulary that supports all efforts to coordinate national preparedness activities.

➤ The *Target Capabilities List* describes 37 specific capabilities (eg, epidemiologic surveillance and outbreak investigation) needed to perform critical homeland security tasks identified in the Universal Task List. The Target Capabilities List is designed to assist local, state, and federal entities understand and define their respective roles in a major event; the capabilities required to perform a specified set of tasks; the people, equipment, and supplies that are needed; and where to obtain additional resources if needed.

Each of these documents can be accessed on the Department of Homeland Security's Lessons Learned Information Sharing Web site at http://www.llis.gov.

Putting NIMS into Practice

The NIMS provides tools to help ensure that government agencies and organizations provide or establish processes for planning, training, and exercising. All jurisdictions can benefit from NIMS by:

➤ Involving all responding agencies, private organizations, and nongovernmental organizations in planning, training, and exercise activities

➤ Integrating the Incident Command System into the jurisdiction's Emergency Operations Plan and procedures

➤ Using the Incident Command System for all incidents, regardless of type

➤ Coordinating the sharing of information and intelligence between the Incident Command and the Emergency Operations Plan or other multiagency coordination entity

➤ Operating as a team, regardless of the agencies or mutual aid partners involved in a response

➤ Communicating among all responding agencies, including mutual aid partners

➤ Maintaining interoperability of all resources, including resources owned by mutual aid partners

➤ Training all personnel who could be involved in a response to minimum proficiency standards

➤ Categorizing all response resources according to performance capability

➤ Identifying, mobilizing, dispatching, tracking, and recovering incident resources

➤ Establishing a Joint Information System to coordinate the release of information to the public

➤ Maintaining complete records of training certifications

➤ Researching and applying best practices from incidents that present the highest risk to their jurisdiction

Source: *National Incident Management System (NIMS), An Introduction*. IS-700 Self-Study Guide; 2004. http://www.training .fema.gov/EMIWeb/downloads/NIMS-Self-Study%20Guide.pdf.

See also *IS-700.a NIMS An Introduction*. http://training.fema.gov/EMIWeb/IS/IS700a.asp.

3.7   ESSENTIALS OF COMMUNITY DISASTER PLANNING

In the event of a catastrophic emergency, community officials will face the challenge of allocating scarce resources to minimize illness, injury, and death. To be better prepared, community plans need to:

➤ *Be created in advance.* Good planning must be done ahead of time. Community planners should consider existing assets and anticipate additional needs and resources (including medical and public health), and identify policy and operational systems to meet these needs.

➤ *Build and maintain relationships.* Community plans should identify partnerships, memoranda of understanding (such as the Emergency Management Assistance Compact), interhospital agreements, and other relationships with key stakeholders from the health care system, emergency management system, state and local public health systems, local emergency responders, EMS, home health care, and other medical providers; volunteer agencies; public safety; and other public and private partners at all government levels. It is paramount that these relationships be maintained to allow for effective coordination when a disaster occurs.

➤ *Establish authorities and responsibilities for emergency actions and the means to garner the resources to support those actions.* Public and private health agencies, facilities, and responders must provide a mechanism for cooperation and coordination of activities, resources, and policy across multiple agencies and jurisdictions. Plans must articulate the chain of command for ensuring leadership and coordination. It is critical to identify the decision-making process for resource allocation and policy guidance.

➤ *Assess the health and safety risks that threaten the jurisdiction with consideration to reducing or eliminating vulnerability.* Local health officials should perform routine epidemiologic surveillance to develop a community health profile with baseline health statistics. Assessments should determine hazards that merit special attention, specific populations that may be at increased risk, what actions must be planned for, what resources are likely to be needed, and the probable impact.

➤ *Establish information dissemination and communications processes.* Clear channels of communication are needed to link the public health community, diverse health care entities, and emergency response systems. This includes mechanisms for sharing accurate, real-time situational information with stakeholders across multiple jurisdictions. Contact information for response components and agencies must be continually updated to allow for timely communication.

➤ *Consider the legal and ethical issues related to disaster planning and response.* Plans must address state emergency powers and the types of events or circumstances that trigger implementation of these powers. Community planners must be familiar with ethical principles that underlie decision making in disasters and public health emergencies, such as for the allocation of scarce resources.

➤ *Consider all populations, including but not limited to those with special needs who may be more vulnerable to adverse health effects.* Explicit planning must occur at all levels for vulnerable populations including infants, children, the frail elderly, pregnant women, the disabled, the mentally ill, and groups with chronic medical conditions or other special medical needs (eg, cardiac, dialysis, and oncology patients). Prior experience has demonstrated that without explicit planning, the needs of these populations will not be adequately met.

➤ *Be exercised and evaluated in realistic scenarios.* Community responders should understand and practice the processes that will be used to work with as well as request resources from each other, from supply vendors,

Elements of a Community Disaster Plan

1. Brief community profile

2. Aims of the plan

3. Hazard vulnerability analysis and risk assessment

4. Resource identification

5. Capability assessment

6. Tasks and responsibilities

7. Concepts of operations and policies

8. Annexes (plan details)

   ➤ Maps, tables, and details (eg, risk assessment, evacuation plan)

   ➤ Directory of organizations and important local government and media contacts

   ➤ Contact list of members of the community disaster management organizations

IMPORTANT POINTS

States and localities vary in size, population, risk, needs, and capabilities, which precludes development of "boilerplate" disaster preparedness and response plans. Plans must consider and accommodate regional and local needs, resources, and capabilities. Disaster plans should:

➤ Be written documents describing who does what

➤ Establish organizational and governmental interrelationships and chain of command

➤ Be all-hazards plans, based on a community risk assessment and the needs of all community populations

➤ Include a mix of short-, medium-, and long-term disaster management activities to reduce vulnerabilities and increase capacities

➤ Identify mechanisms and timelines for conducting community drills or disaster simulation exercises

➤ Provide mechanisms for periodic review and ongoing improvement, as well as mechanisms for informing all stakeholders of the revisions/changes

and from emergency management contacts. Community disaster plans should be evaluated continually through tabletop exercises and full-scale drills, involving all key stakeholders, including local hospitals, businesses, and schools. Opportunities such as special events (eg, major sporting events, political conventions) can be used to test disaster plans.

Community disaster plans address the short- and long-term objectives of preparedness, response, and recovery activities to include mobilization of resources to protect public health and safety; restoration of essential government services;

FIGURE 3-2

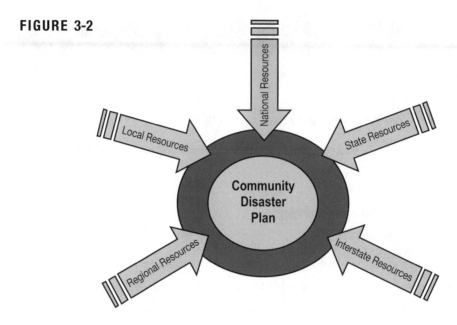

and provision of emergency relief to government, businesses, and victims. Well-coordinated plans are essential for the mobilization of assets from local, regional, and national sources in a predetermined manner (Figure 3-2).

3.7.1   Pre-event Planning

Mitigation planning aims to lessen the severity and impact of a potential emergency. It involves reducing exposure to, probability of, or potential loss from hazardous events. This includes zoning and building code requirements and strategies for educating businesses and the public on measures they can take to reduce loss and injury (such as fastening bookshelves, water heaters, and file cabinets to walls to keep them from falling during an earthquake).

Preparedness planning involves the development of the resources and organizational capacity to prevent or manage the effects of a disaster on the basis of local risk assessments. The PRE-DISASTER Paradigm™ (Planning and practice, Resilience, Education) emphasizes the actions to build preparedness. Preparedness involves all of the actions required in advance to establish and sustain the level of capability necessary to execute a wide range of disaster management operations involving the public and private sectors. Preparedness plans describe how personnel, equipment, and other governmental and nongovernmental resources will be used to support incident management requirements. Plans provide mechanisms for setting priorities, integrating multiple entities and functions, requesting disaster assistance from state and federal authorities, establishing collaborative relationships, and ensuring that communications and other systems support the complete spectrum of incident management activities.

Local health officials should work with other stakeholders to integrate and coordinate regional and community disaster preparedness plans. This involves:

➤ Conducting disaster training and education

➤ Mapping specific locations of potential disasters

➤ Performing hazard vulnerability and risk assessments

➤ Taking inventory of existing health resources and assessing the ability to mobilize those resources in an emergency (ie, surge capacity planning)

➤ Designating alternate care facilities and shelters

➤ Providing medical and mental health services, including procedures for meeting community needs when local resources are overwhelmed, damaged, or disrupted

➤ Providing mechanisms for managing and distributing inventories of countermeasures that might be needed for various threat scenarios (eg, if mass clinics are needed, thousands of volunteers will be required, preferably coming from organized volunteer groups)

Risk assessment is an important component of disaster preparedness planning. It is a participatory process to identify and assess hazards that threaten the community with corresponding assessment of community vulnerabilities and capacities. The process begins by conducting a *hazard vulnerability analysis*, which identifies potential hazards that may affect local operations. Strategies need to be developed to address perceived vulnerabilities that are most likely to occur. Types of hazards include, but are not limited to:

➤ Public utility disruptions (extended power interruptions)

➤ Infrastructure damage (bridge or building collapse)

➤ Communicable disease outbreaks

➤ Natural disasters (eg, tornados, hurricanes, earthquakes, floods)

➤ Fire

➤ Hazardous material spills

➤ Industrial plant explosions

➤ Terrorist attacks

➤ Civil disorder

3.7.2 Postevent Planning

Response planning deals with how local agencies and organizations will be engaged and mobilized when a disaster occurs. After a disaster occurs, planning must address the possible consequences to the government, businesses, and affected populations by protecting public health and safety, restoring essential

Elements of a Community Risk Assessment

Community risk assessment involves four interrelated components:

➤ *Risk perception:* understanding how different people perceive and measure risk

➤ *Hazard assessment:* analyzing various hazards for a particular geographic area and the magnitude of impact given local resources, allowing for prioritization of response and mitigation options

➤ *Vulnerability assessment:* identifying particular infrastructures and populations at increased risk for damage or harm

➤ *Capacity assessment:* identifying available resources that can be used to reduce risk, enhance survival, and help affected individuals and populations cope with severe trauma

It is important to understand the difference between the terms *risk* and *hazard*. A *hazard* is anything that has the potential to do harm to property, the environment, people, or animals. *Risk* is the probability of the potential hazard actually occurring.

---

government services, and providing emergency relief. Community resources will likely be challenged by a surge of people seeking treatment, prophylaxis, or decontamination, as well as shelter and food. Linking people to medical services in an emergency must be coordinated with area hospitals, clinics, urgent care facilities, and private health care facilities. Effective, efficient communication plans are key to getting the word out to the general public about these resources.

To effectively implement the planned response to the disaster, the responsible government entities must be capable and able to respond. That is, they must have sufficient continuity of government operations and resources so that they may direct the response and are capable of requesting assistance from external sources when the infrastructure of the government agency is destroyed by the disaster.

Response planning involves consideration of time-sensitive actions to save lives and property, as well as actions to begin stabilizing the situation to help the community cope with the situation. These include:

➤ Implementation of incident management systems

➤ Mobilization and coordination of community resources for emergency response (coordination of search and rescue, triage, decontamination, and emergency medical care)

➤ Casualty distribution

➤ Management of volunteers and donations

➤ Provision of disaster relief and assistance to victims

➤ Notification procedures to alert emergency response personnel to the crisis, and a means to request help from outside entities

➤ Protection of emergency responders

➤ Public health intervention (eg, surveillance)

➤ Evacuation or sheltering of populations, as appropriate

➤ Food handling, mass feeding, and sanitation services in emergency facilities

➤ Support for emergency personnel (food, shelter, sanitation)

➤ Public information dissemination and mass media involvement

Recovery planning addresses continuity of operations, the restoration of essential services and infrastructure, and resumption of normal social and economic activities with minimal delay. This includes the reestablishment of necessary public utilities and services (eg, power, communication, water and sewage, transportation, law enforcement), providing for basic human needs (eg, food, clothing, and shelter), and ensuring that the health and social needs of affected individuals are met (eg, provision of medical and mental health services). Recovery planning also includes mechanisms to evaluate disaster response to improve future efforts.

3.8 COMMUNITY PLANNING FOR A PANDEMIC[13-15]

A *pandemic* is a new infectious disease that emerges to which the population has little or no immunity. This lack of immunity allows it to spread rapidly across the population. An influenza pandemic or other large-scale infectious disease outbreak has the potential to cause widespread illness and death throughout the world and is an example of a public health emergency that can severely challenge community preparedness planning efforts. Although the timing, nature, and severity of a pandemic cannot be predicted with any certainty, community preparedness planning is imperative to lessen the impact of the event. The unique characteristics and events of a pandemic will strain local, state, and federal resources. It is unlikely that there will be sufficient personnel, equipment, and supplies to respond adequately to multiple areas of the country for a sustained period of time. Therefore, minimizing social and economic disruption will require a coordinated response. Governments, communities, and other public and private sector stakeholders will need to anticipate and prepare for a pandemic by defining roles and responsibilities and developing continuity of operations plans.

The ubiquitous nature of an influenza pandemic compels federal, state, and local governments, communities, corporations, families, and individuals to learn about, prepare for, and collaborate in efforts to mitigate, slow, respond to, and recover from this disease. The development, refinement, and practicing of pandemic influenza plans by all stakeholders are critical components of preparedness. Because an influenza pandemic has the capacity to cause disruptions across all levels of government in all communities, pandemic influenza preparedness is a responsibility shared by government, public health, and heatlh care organizations.

Three influenza pandemics occurred in the past century: two as recently as 1968 and 1957 and one in 1918, in which what has been called the Great Influenza pandemic killed 40 to 50 million people worldwide. In spring 2009, a novel H1N1 influenza A virus emerged and spread rapidly, creating a widespread outbreak of the disease. In June 2009, the World Health Organization (WHO) declared the existence of global pandemic. Adequate planning for and response to this situation requires the involvement of all levels of government and indeed, the world. Plans of the US Department of Health and Human Services,[14] WHO,[15] and others are focused on bringing the H1N1 influenza pandemic under control as rapidly as possible. State pandemic plans can be found at http://pandemicflu.gov/professional/states/index.html#stateinfo.

3.8.1   Containment

Containment refers to the WHO plan to define and contain the outbreak in specific geographic regions. This is an aggressive proactive plan to isolate individuals and communities that are infected with the virus to help prevent the spread of the virus. Even if not fully successful, containment decisions can help slow the spread of the virus, allowing additional time for implementation of other control measures.

In a pandemic or other serious public health emergency, public health officials have authority to implement various measures to control the spread of the disease. This includes issuing travel advisories, imposing border restrictions, and restricting domestic and global travel. Planning for restrictions on international travel might be considered necessary, depending on the properties of the virus and the location of the outbreak. Persons who limit their own personal risk by canceling nonessential trips will help control disease spread. Limiting or canceling travel of US residents and others from affected countries will depend on the properties of the pandemic virus that emerges and will be informed by the facts at the time.

3.8.2   Coordinated Communication and Information Sharing

Controlling a pandemic requires a coordinated communications plan involving global, federal, state, and local authorities and the public. Access to accurate and reliable information will be critical. This includes announcements to advise health professionals and the public on the best course of action by means of multiple media venues throughout different phases of the pandemic. Health messages should stress the importance of prevention and personal hygiene as the most basic and most important way to prevent the spread of the virus. This includes frequent handwashing and proper cough etiquette (ie, covering the mouth and nose with a tissue when coughing or sneezing, coughing or sneezing into the elbow instead of the hands), avoiding close contact with sick people, and the appropriate use of personal protective equipment such as surgical masks or N95 respirators (close-fitting masks that filter at least 95% of airborne particles).

Pandemic plans also specify how local health authorities will work with clinicians and community leaders to implement alternate care facilities, dedicated community hotlines, and information systems. Persons who are ill or have been exposed to someone who is ill may be advised to call the hotline for information about the disease and treatment options.

3.8.3   Social Distancing

A pandemic influenza virus spreads only through human-to-human contact. To prevent infection, public health authorities will plan for the implementation of "social distancing" rules. *Social distancing* is an important disease prevention strategy in which a community imposes limitations on social (face-to-face) interactions to reduce exposure to and transmission of the virus. These limitations could include, but are not restricted to, facility closures, telecommuting, cancellation of public gatherings, and shutting down mass transportation. Experience with past flu pandemics has shown that limiting contact among people during the outbreak can help slow the spread of the virus and save lives.

Possible social distancing measures include:

➤ Closing schools and child care programs, canceling school-based activities, and limiting opportunities for out-of-school social interaction

➤ Limiting contact in the community and workplace through cancellation of public gatherings, conferences, and business meetings, and restricting travel. Employers and employees will need to plan for possible changes in work schedules and business operations including telecommuting.

In a flu pandemic, most sick people will be asked to stay home and will be given instructions for taking care of themselves. Sick persons may be advised to avoid going to the hospital unless they have severe respiratory problems or other serious symptoms as defined by health authorities. Family members also may be asked to stay home if a person in the household is sick, because they could spread the virus to others.

3.8.4 Mass Prophylaxis and Care

Public health authorities are responsible for developing community plans and strategies for the care of sick, exposed, and dead persons. This includes the following:

➤ *Issuing guidance for the diagnosis, care, and reporting of sick persons.* Health officials will provide guidelines for the distribution of scarce medical resources to those who need and/or can benefit from them most, and for the isolation and treatment of all persons with confirmed or probable pandemic influenza. Isolation of sick persons may occur in the home or health care setting, depending on the severity of the person's illness and/or the capacity of the health care system to provide such care. Consideration will be given to providing sufficient quantities of effective medications, as appropriate, and ensuring that there is a feasible way of distributing these medications to homebound persons.

➤ *Distributing medications to large numbers of the population, including determining the locations of mass vaccination and treatment clinics and how to staff such clinics.* A basic part of a large-scale outbreak or pandemic would be setting up dispensing sites for distributing antibiotics or providing vaccinations or other medications. The number of sites should be scalable depending on the anticipated need. While planning includes identifying and training site volunteers and staff before an event, there should also be refresher and "just-in-time" training available before administering prophylaxis to the public. There are roles for both medical and nonmedical volunteers.

➤ *Coordinating efforts to manage potentially large numbers of persons who die from the disease.*

Early in the pandemic, a vaccine will probably not be available for the new influenza virus. The major changes that have occurred in the virus mean existing vaccines will have limited to no effectiveness. Prescribed medications such as antivirals may not be effective and may be in limited quantities. Public health officials will work to develop a national stockpile of antiviral drugs to help treat and control the spread of the disease and support the production and testing of possible vaccines, including finding more reliable and quicker ways to make large quantities of vaccines.

In a pandemic, physicians and other health care professionals need to be prepared to shift their usual practice of devoting much attention to the most critically ill to (1) helping those who are most likely to survive with the scarcity of resources available and (2) preventing others from being infected. This shift in clinical decision making will come from a central and local public health authority and will be implemented in all health facilities and hospital systems.

3.9 DISASTER PLANNING FOR HOSPITALS AND THE HEALTH CARE SECTOR

Health facility disaster planning is a component of larger community planning and, therefore, requires coordination with other local entities. Facility plans need to be developed in partnership with community groups, including law enforcement, fire safety, public health, EMS, and pediatric and mental health professionals. The extent to which these various groups interface varies by region and whether the incident is of local, state, or national significance.

At the institutional level, the development of external and internal emergency plans should be considered. An *external disaster* is anything that indirectly affects an institution's infrastructure. This type of event in the health care sector would address how to manage an increased number of patients for triage, decontamination, transport, and treatment. An *internal disaster* plan includes conditions that affect a facility directly (such a building fire) and may be an extension of an external emergency. This type of disaster carries the additional burden of not just caring for patients but also ensuring the safety of patients and staff. Disaster planning must address the possibility that the health care facility itself becomes a disaster "victim" and is unable to provide care. The Joint Commission now requires that hospitals be self-sufficient in their emergency management for a minimum of 72 hours, with a goal of 96 hours.

3.9.1 Capacity Assessment

When developing a facility disaster plan, it is essential to assess existing capacity in each of the following four categories[16]:

➤ Existing plans and policies

➣ Fire/flood protection plan

➣ Facility security procedures

➣ Insurance polices

➣ Finance and purchasing procedures

➣ Employee policies

➣ Risk management plan

➤ Personnel

➣ Total number of staff, including skill sets

➣ Total number of staff available in an emergency

> Staff potentially vulnerable during an emergency (eg, due to limited physical ability)

> Proximity of staff to the facility

➤ Equipment

> Fire protection and suppression equipment

> Communications equipment

> First aid and triage supplies

> Emergency power equipment

> Personal protective equipment

> Decontamination capability

➤ Backup systems for critical functions/continuity of operations

> Offsite storage of paper or electronic medical records

> Payroll

> Communications

> Patient services

> Computer systems

Effective emergency preparedness in health care facilities also requires planning for large-scale events that affect many people. These events may include chemical, biologic, radiation, or natural disasters. A critical component of the ability to respond to large-scale disasters is surge capacity.[17-19] In addition to assessment of existing capacity, it is essential that health care facilities also assess their ability to respond effectively to a mass influx of patients, which may disrupt daily operations. *Surge capacity* is the ability of a health care system to rapidly expand beyond normal services to meet the increased demand for care of patients. This surge occurs in physical space/hospital beds, qualified personnel, medical care, and public health services in the event of a large-scale disaster or public health emergency.

3.9.2   Health Facility Planning Considerations[1,16,20,21]

In the event of a catastrophic emergency, health facility officials (like community officials) will face the challenge of allocating scarce resources to minimize illness, injury, and death. To meet this challenge, facility disaster plans should:

➤ *Be developed with input from staff members from various levels and departments.* The disaster team should work together to formulate the plan, train employees, and supervise drills. Planning for and meeting the challenges of disasters and other serious emergencies requires leadership. The disaster team must be prepared and empowered to make decisions. Distributing authority across a prepared team will improve the quality of the response.

➤ *Address the types of emergencies most relevant to the facility, its geographic location, and the needs of the individuals and patient community served.* Facility disaster plans must be realistic, tailored to local needs, and up to date at all times. While it is important that a disaster plan be broad enough to address all possible hazards, the planning team should determine the most likely risks for the region and give particular attention to these in the plan. Is the facility in a flood zone or hurricane-prone area? Does the plan include procedures for power outages during extreme temperatures? Disaster plans will differ between jurisdictions because the potential hazards, laws, and resources will vary.

➤ *Involve local emergency management authorities.* Local emergency planning officials should be consulted to ensure that the plan does not conflict with the city or county plan. City or county emergency planning staff can help identify local disaster risks and resources. Working with local officials of government, law enforcement, utilities, schools, and community organizations will help to coordinate emergency responses.

To address environmental disasters such as toxic spills, hurricanes, tornadoes, floods, and earthquakes, local institutions should consult with the local community planning infrastructure, such as local emergency planning committees. These groups identify and catalog potential hazards and resources to mitigate disasters, when feasible, and write emergency plans. The local emergency planning infrastructure can work with local hospitals, schools, and businesses to address environmental hazards or vulnerabilities and provide resources for examining potential risks.

➤ *Delineate policies and procedures to independently manage essential health, safety, and personal needs of patients and staff.* A health facility disaster plan should provide for sources of emergency utilities and supplies, including gas, water, food, and essential medical supplies and equipment. Hospitals and other health care facilities need to assess their current capacity and develop a plan to achieve surge capacity. Plans and procedures need to be in place for controlling facility air flow and ventilation systems to prevent or limit dispersal of airborne contaminants. In a large-scale disaster, individuals should plan to be self-sufficient for a minimum of 72 hours, with a goal of 96 hours. The number of days the facility's backup generator can supply electrical power and the elevation of emergency generators in relation to flood planning should be taken into account. Many hospitals have generators that are located in their basement, making them useless during a flood event. Consideration also needs to be given to:

➢ Triage, decontamination, use of personal protective equipment, and infection control

➢ Provision of essential medications and medical supplies

> ➤ Adequate food and water for patients and staff who will be required to stay at the facility, as well as for others, particularly staff and family of staff, who may use the facility for shelter

> ➤ Systems to prepare, serve, and store food in the event of a power outage

> ➤ Systems and supplies for the use of alternative water sources including the purification of water if potable water is lost, and a method to transport water from its source to patient care areas

> ➤ Systems and supplies to maintain a minimum standard of hygiene and sanitation

➤ *Describe procedures for assigning and recalling staff and chart the facility's lines of authority.* The Hospital Incident Command System provides an orderly and efficient chain of command and job action sheets to simplify this need. An efficient emergency response requires that everyone be clear about what their assignment is and who is in charge. Regulations require each facility to delineate internal lines of authority in a disaster. Staff members need to know what is expected regarding "call backs" or "holdovers" at work during an emergency. Communicating this expectation ahead of time allows them to prepare their family emergency plan accordingly. Telephones, including cellular telephones, may not be functional during the first few hours or days after a disaster, so predetermined arrangements for staff to report to work and alternative communication plans are important. Familiarity with the hospital incident command system is helpful.

➤ *Address internal and external evacuation policies and procedures.* Some emergencies require full patient evacuation and transfer. Plans should consider quick evacuation in case of facility fire or collapse, as well as mass transfer to alternate facilities. Plans should outline procedures for emergency transfer of patients who can be moved to other health facilities, including arrangements for safe and efficient transportation. Evacuation routes and strategies need to be planned.

➤ *Plan for transportation needs and discuss these plans with local emergency management officials to ensure they do not conflict with existing agreements or plans.* The plan should include safe procedures for the movement and housing of patients within the facility, as well as how tasks, such as food preparation and hygiene, will be managed in areas that may not be designed for such activities. In addition, health facility plans should address procedures for the emergency discharge of patients, including arrangements for their care, transportation, and follow-up.

➤ *Define procedures for maintaining a record of patient movement and a method of sending all pertinent personal and medical information with patients, so that an accurate record can be maintained of when and where they went.* Patients should be accompanied by a record containing basic medical information including medications, diet, and medical conditions as well as personal information relevant to their care. This is especially critical for patients who cannot communicate their medical care needs. To prepare for any emergency, systems should be in place for backup, storage, and retrieval of important patient and employee information.

➤ *Establish reciprocal or other agreements with nearby facilities to provide temporary care.* Prior arrangements should be made with nearby hospitals to transfer patients safely and efficiently if the facility becomes disabled or unsafe for patients. The plan should include provisions for the conversion of usable space for the immediate care of emergency admissions. If the facility is not directly impacted by the disaster, it may be used to provide shelter and care for others. Provisions in the facility plan must address how emergency admissions will be managed in an orderly manner. Consideration should be given to the use of schools as alternate care facilities by providing space (eg, shelter, temporary clinics, morgues) and supplies (eg, school meal diversion) for the community during a crisis.

➤ *Address employee communications.* Employees should be given emergency telephone numbers of physicians, health facilities, and local fire and EMS responders, as well as processes for notifying family members, guardians, or others responsible for patient welfare. Staff must act quickly during a disaster, and the information they need should be up-to-date and included in the facility's plan. A plan should be created to communicate with employees, suppliers, community leaders, and the public. Staff may need to report to work immediately or be notified to report to an alternative care facility.

Facility staff need to work with local emergency officials to address the use of a shared incident command vocabulary and ensure that communication systems and devices can be aligned so that fire, police, and other community officials are on the same radio frequency. Staff should learn how to access and utilize multiple communication options, while realizing that they may not have the ability to communicate with everyone.

➤ *Address public communications.* A spokesperson should be designated to provide official statements to the media. Assigning an individual who is skilled in communication and prepared to deal with inquiries from the public and the media is essential in preventing the spread of misinformation.

➤ *Delineate security policies and procedures.* During the aftermath of Hurricane Katrina, some hospitals were overpowered by desperate and hungry residents seeking food, shelter, and other necessities. Health facility officials should work with community leaders to determine the types of emergencies for which the facility will provide nonpatient community services. Arrangements should be made with local law enforcement officials and private security firms to provide security reinforcements as needed.

During a disaster, many people may come to the facility looking for medical assistance. Relatives and family members also may arrive to check on loved ones. Staff need to know how to keep unauthorized individuals out of the facility and how to manage concerned family members. Additionally, it is important that staff have appropriate identification to allow them to cross a police or fire barrier should the area be restricted.

➤ *Be reviewed and practiced continually.* The plan should be evaluated often and modified as needed. All staff members must know the location of the facility plan and receive ongoing education and training for implementing the plan. New employees should be oriented to the plan at the time they begin employment and annually thereafter.

The facility should comply with all applicable regulations for disaster drills (such as those of the Joint Commission and the Occupational Safety and Health Administration). Health care facilities should participate in state and local disaster drills when asked by emergency management authorities. Disaster drills and exercises should be used not only to practice the facility plan, but as a way to identify opportunities for improvement. A written report of all drills and exercises should be generated, and if problems are identified, follow-up action must be documented. Even though a health facility may never experience a serious disaster, it will likely encounter circumstances that will test the emergency plan. Health facility officials should learn from those experiences.

3.10 PLANNING FOR THE NEEDS OF VULNERABLE POPULATIONS

While the disaster health system seeks to prevent and control injuries and disease in all populations, particular attention is directed to those with special health needs. In the aftermath of Hurricane Katrina, various health-related needs and issues surfaced at a magnitude not previously experienced by state and local health officials.[3,22-24] Traditional response and recovery operations could not meet all of the resulting human needs, in either the short or the long term. Addressing the great diversity of special health concerns, language and cultural barriers, and other life circumstances presented multiple challenges for disaster response and recovery systems.

The terms *special needs* and *vulnerable populations* refer to many different groups of people in the community. For the National Disaster Life Support™ Program, these terms are used interchangeably to characterize groups whose needs are not fully addressed by traditional service providers. These are populations who cannot comfortably or safely access and use the medical and mental health resources that are offered through community preparedness, response, and recovery operations. Vulnerable populations include, but are not limited to, those who are physically or mentally disabled (blind, deaf, hard-of-hearing, or having cognitive disorders or mobility limitations), those with limited English or non-English speaking, those who are geographically or culturally isolated, those who are medically or chemically dependent, the homeless, the frail elderly, pregnant women, and children.

Situations and circumstances that may render persons to be especially vulnerable in a disaster include:

> *Being dependent on support services.* People who depend on other persons or community support services to perform daily activities may be more vulnerable when their "lifelines" are disrupted. This may include a disabled person whose needs cannot be met in a shelter or a frail elderly person who lives alone and has limited mobility.

> *Living in high-risk areas.* People who live in older or lower-income neighborhoods may be more vulnerable to structural damage from disasters.

> *Having limited access to community services.* People who lack resources, trust, knowledge, or ability to access community services and systems may have greater difficulty preparing for, responding to, and recovering from disasters.

> *Having limited economic resources and social support systems.* People lacking money, education, employment, or other resources and support systems are likely to have fewer coping mechanisms with which to recover from a disaster. This may include a non–English-speaking person who does not understand a mandatory evacuation order or a recent immigrant who is reluctant to ask for help.

Populations That May Have Special Health Needs in a Disaster
➤ Frail elderly
➤ People with disabilities, chronic medical conditions, and mental health problems
➤ Children
➤ Pregnant women
➤ Non–English-speaking persons
➤ People who are culturally or geographically isolated
➤ People with substance abuse problems
➤ People who are homeless, marginally housed, or shelter-dependent
➤ People living in poverty

People with special health needs must be identified and have valid emergency care plans in place, including plans for managing day-to-day problems related to their specific illness or disability, as well as plans for managing health-related needs in the event of a disaster or public health emergency. In a large-scale emergency, medical supplies and equipment may be limited. During a prolonged lockdown or shelter-in-place situation, the availability of medications can pose a serious challenge for persons with chronic diseases.

3.11   COMMUNICATING IN A DISASTER[1,3,5,25]

The criticality of a disaster situation includes the potential of dramatically increased utilization of communications media. Anxious family members will overwhelm telephone lines with calls in the event of a serious incident involving mass casualties. Health and emergency response agencies will require ongoing open external and internal communication channels. The ability to establish and maintain open lines for efficient communication with health care facilities, emergency workers, and public safety organizations is critical.

3.11.1   Emergency Communication Planning

A carefully prepared plan is needed to protect vital communication links among all emergency responders and ensure that information interchange can continue. All agencies that may respond to a disaster in a community must cooperate in advance to identify those methods of communication that will persist under most conceivable conditions. In a disaster, the ability to establish and maintain open lines to communicate efficiently with health care facilities, public health agencies, emergency management agencies, public safety organizations, and citizens is crucial. All emergency responders must be able to communicate effectively with one another multidirectionally, in real time, using a common language, before, during, and after the event occurs. Information and communication networks should be redundant, secure, and linked to the public health and health care systems for disease surveillance and timely information sharing. The NIMS prescribes interoperable communications systems for both incident and information management to standardize communications during a disaster.

Telephone communications systems (cellular and landline) often become overwhelmed during a disaster because of the number of people who are using the system to communicate with family members to ascertain their well-being or to inform others of the event. Emergency planners, responders, and health care providers should enroll in the Government Emergency Telecommunications System (GETS). This system allows users to dial a code that will override system congestion and receive priority routing of telephone calls to ensure that they will be able to communicate during the disaster or public health emergency. The cellular system is referred to as GETS-WPS (Wireless Priority Service). See the GETS Web site at http://gets.ncs.gov/ for information on the GETS.

Storms or earthquakes may knock out power lines, disrupting telephone services, radio and television stations, and possibly even dispatch agencies. Scenario testing of potential losses of communication should be conducted to predict how municipalities would handle the various communication needs should the transfer of information be temporarily disabled or even destroyed. Communities should plan to have at least two or more appropriate, proven communication systems, at least one of which is "hardened" to be available in virtually any disaster. A hardened response might be, for example, the rapid deployment of the Radio Amateur Civil Emergency Service (RACES) under standing orders from the fire chief of the community to call a neighboring fire department to place a call for emergency assistance or mutual aid, to notify surrounding hospital facilities, and perhaps even to contact the military for assistance.

Disaster communication plans must be based on a clear understanding of the needs and perceptions of the target audience. This includes systems and protocols for communicating timely and accurate information to the public. Strategies need to consider how to reach persons of different cultures, races, and religions, as well as meet the needs of disabled (eg, blind, hearing impaired) and disenfranchised (eg, homeless, impoverished) persons.

During emergencies, the public may receive information from a variety of sources. Effective communication of clear, concise, and credible information will help ensure the public that the situation is being addressed competently. Under NIMS, state and local health authorities must have established procedures for providing the news media with timely and accurate public information. One way to ensure coordination of public information is by establishing a Joint Information Center (JIC). Using the JIC as a central location, information can be coordinated and integrated across jurisdictions and agencies, and among all government partners, the private sector, and nongovernmental agencies.

Communicating with the Public in a Disaster

Disaster communications should be developed with the following considerations:

➤ Response should be quick and accurate. In a crisis, the first 24 hours are critical. If the facts and the implications of those facts are not provided, the media and public will speculate and form opinions on their own.

➤ A primary person should be identified to be the "voice" of the agency or organization. The public must receive a single, clear message. Multiple voices, even when delivering the same information, may be perceived as conveying different messages.

➤ During communication, the nature of the content that is released must be carefully controlled. The individual communicating with the media must always tell the truth but should resist giving every detail.

➤ The message relayed to the media must be one of concern, compassion, and understanding. The authorized individual communicating with the media must not panic, especially under media pressure.

➤ Communications should avoid the use of "factoid" sound bites that sound good but have no ultimate consequences.

➤ The role and efforts of the media in emergency management should be recognized and appreciated.

3.11.2   Communication Modalities

While calls for help commonly come from landline telephones, the growing use of cellular telephones clearly indicates that they will become the preferred method of notification and activation of emergency response systems. Thus, "enhanced 911" systems must be modified to allow for "wireless enhanced 911" ability to localize callers in emergency settings.

Given the common dependence of municipal agencies on cellular telephones, it is clear that restrictions must be placed, in advance, on cellular telephone channels to suppress unnecessary use of specific channels and ensure access to municipal agencies. Likewise, emergency radio channels must be strictly protected for the use of involved disaster response personnel.

Widespread access to the Internet has made detailed information for managing virtually any emergency readily available. The Health Alert Network was developed by the Centers for Disease Control and Prevention (CDC) to facilitate rapid dissemination of essential information to front-line health care and public health workers about disease outbreaks and other public health emergencies.[26] Such information can assist health care professionals in making diagnoses and instituting proper infection control measures to prevent disease spread.

Alternate communication systems may be used if the power is disrupted or the landline telephones are inoperable. The increased use of cellular telephones can overwhelm system capacities. Citizen band, ham radio, two-way radios (walkie-talkies), and satellite systems also should be considered. In severe situations, word of mouth and hand-painted signs may be necessary.

Direct satellite telecommunication devices or microwave uplinks also can be used in disaster situations. An example of such an uplink is the establishment of direct Internet communication for tracking victims, allocating resources, and providing information. Municipal trials with such satellite uplinks are ongoing and have shown promise, mirroring similar devices used by the military (eg, instant worldwide medical record availability on armed service personnel who become ill or injured during a military maneuver).

In addition, mobile data terminals and personal digital assistants (PDAs) have an important role in disaster management. Sophisticated PDA software can provide comprehensive patient treatment algorithms, pharmacology information, and toxicology references for emergency responders and hospital medical staff. Such resources may be extremely

---

CDC Clinician Outreach and Communication

The CDC provides a free registry to provide clinicians with real-time information to help prepare for (and possibly respond to) terrorism and other emergency events. Participants receive regular e-mail updates on terrorism and other relevant emergency issues and training opportunities. See http://www.bt.cdc.gov/clinregistry/index.asp.

useful in biologic, chemical, or radiation emergencies in which the provider lacks recent experience or familiarity with this type of situation.

Other communications technologies available to public health and emergency medical responders include automated callouts, simple voice mail, or automatic call forwarding to another location. Many communities, for example, are capable of making "reverse 911" calls. This provides the Emergency Operations Center with the ability to send telephone messages to landline and cellular telephones within the geographic area at risk. The system is designed to provide map- or list-based communications with key audiences. Geographic calling zones are created on the basis of immediate circumstances or in advance on the basis of anticipated needs.

Modes of Communication in a Disaster

Modes of communication that can be considered in reaching diverse populations include:

➤ Telephone-based communication

  ➣ Fixed-line telephone systems

  ➣ Cellular (mobile) telephone systems

  ➣ Private electronic mail (e-mail) and text messaging

  ➣ Satellite systems

➤ Public meetings, briefings

➤ National and local television networks

  ➣ Internet-based communication Web sites

  ➣ E-mail

  ➣ Blogs and social networking sites (eg, Twitter, Facebook, MySpace)

➤ Radio-based communication

  ➣ Radio communication via police, fire, EMS, and ambulance services

  ➣ Amateur radio networks (eg, ham radio, RACES)

  ➣ Community-based and broadcast radio stations

  ➣ Satellite radio

➤ Print communications

  ➣ Newspapers

  ➣ Community mailings (eg, flyers and newsletters)

3.12   SUMMARY

To effectively prepare for and respond to an actual or threatened emergency, health officials and other emergency management personnel must collaborate in the development of comprehensive community and institutional plans that:

➤ Identify the types of events that are most likely to affect the community, business, or institution.

➤ Delineate and test emergency response actions and activities in advance to ensure a coordinated response to the consequences of credible threats.

➤ Build the capabilities and capacities necessary to respond effectively to the consequence of those events.

➤ Implement the planned response quickly and efficiently.

➤ Mobilize resources to recover from the incident.

Community disaster plans address the short- and long-term objectives of preparedness, response, and recovery activities to include mobilization of resources to protect public health and safety; restoration of essential government services; and provision of emergency relief to government, businesses, and victims. Well-coordinated plans are essential for the mobilization of assets from local, regional, and national sources in a predetermined manner.

States and localities vary in size, population, risk, needs, and capabilities, which precludes development of "boilerplate" disaster preparedness and response plans. Plans must consider and accommodate regional and local needs, resources, and capabilities.

3.13   SELF-LEARNING SCENARIOS

After completing the CDLS course and each of the chapters in this manual, take time to work through the 4 scenarios presented in Appendix A. The scenarios are designed for the application and reinforcement of "core" concepts and principles in disaster life support.

REFERENCES

1. Landesman LY. *Public Health Management of Disasters: The Practice Guide.* 2nd ed. Washington, DC: American Public Health Association; 2005.

2. Centers for Disease Control and Prevention. *Public Health Emergency Response Guide for State, Local and Tribal Public Health Directors.* Version 1.0. http://emergency.cdc.gov /planning/pdf/cdcresponseguide.pdf. Accessed June 30, 2009.

3. Federal Emergency Management Agency and Department of Homeland Security Office for Civil Rights and Civil Liberties. *Interim Emergency Management Planning Guide for Special Needs Populations. Comprehensive* Preparedness *Guide (CPG) 301*. Version 1.0. Washington, DC: FEMA; 2008. http://www.fema.gov/pdf/media/2008/301.pdf. Accessed June 30, 2009.

4. Phillip SJ, Knebel A, eds. *Mass Medical Care With Scarce Resources: A Community Planning Guide*. Publication 07-0001. Rockville, MD: Agency for Healthcare Research and Quality; 2007. http://www.ahrq.gov/research/mce/. Accessed June 30, 2009.

5. Federal Emergency Management Agency. *Developing and Maintaining State, Territorial, Tribal, and Local Government Plans (Comprehensive Preparedness Guide 101)*. Washington, DC: FEMA; 2009. http://www.fema.gov/pdf/about/divisions/npd/cpg_101 _layout.pdf. Accessed June 30, 2009.

6. Homeland Security Presidential Directive 21 (HSPD-21). Washington, DC: The White House, 2007. http://www.fas.org/irp/offdocs/nspd/hspd-21.htm. Accessed October 23, 2009.

7. *Biodefense for the 21st Century*. www.dhs.gov/xlibrary/assets/HSPD10Biodefensefor21st Century042804.pdf. Accessed January 6, 2009.

8. US Department of Homeland Security. *National Preparedness Guidelines*. Washington, DC: US Department of Homeland Security; 2007. http://www.dhs.gov/xlibrary/assets/ National_Preparedness_Guidelines.pdf. Accessed June 30, 2009.

9. US Department of Homeland Security. *National Response Framework*. Washington, DC: US Department of Homeland Security; 2008. http://www.fema.gov/pdf/emergency/nrf/nrf-core. pdf. Accessed June 30, 2009.

10. Homeland Presidential Security Directive 5 (HSPD-5). Washington, DC: The White House, 2003. http://www.fas.org/irp/offdocs/nspd/hspd-5.html. Accessed June 30, 2009.

11. Federal Emergency Management Agency. NIMS resource center. Washington, DC: FEMA; 2009. http://www.fema.gov/emergency/nims/. Accessed June 30, 2009.

12. Homeland Security Directive 8: National Preparedness. Washington, DC: The White House, 2003. http://www.dhs.gov/xabout/laws/gc_1215444247124.shtm. Accessed June 30, 2009.

13. Knobler SL, Mack A, Mahmoud A, Lemon SM, eds. *The Threat of Pandemic Influenza: Are We Ready? A Workshop Report*. Washington, DC: National Academies Press; 2005.

14. *HHS Pandemic Influenza Plan*. Washington, DC: US Department of Health and Human Services; 2005. http://www.hhs.gov/pandemicflu/plan/pdf/HHSPandemicInfluenzaPlan.pdf. Accessed June 30, 2009.

15. World Health Organization. *Pandemic Influenza Preparedness and Response: a WHO Guidance Document*. Geneva, Switzerland: WHO; 2009. http://www.who.int/csr/ disease/influenza/PIPGuidance09.pdf. Accessed June 30, 2009.

16. Center for Health Policy and the New York Consortium for Emergency Preparedness Continuing Education. *Emergency Preparedness Toolkit for Office-Based Health Care Practices*. New York, NY: Columbia University School of Nursing; 2008.

17. Agency for Healthcare Research and Quality. *Optimizing Surge Capacity: Hospital Assessment and Planning*. Issue Brief No. 3. AHRQ publication 04-P008. Washington, DC: AHRQ; 2004. http://archive.ahrq.gov/news/ulp/btbriefs/btbrief3.htm. Accessed October 20, 2009.

18. Agency for Healthcare Research and Quality. *Addressing Surge Capacity in a Mass Casualty Event*. Issue Brief No. 9. AHRQ publication 06-0027. Washington, DC: AHRQ; 2006. http://archive.ahrq.gov/news/ulp/btbriefs/btbrief9.htm. Accessed October 20, 2009.

19. National Center for Injury Prevention and Control. *In a Moment's Notice: Surge Capacity for Terrorist Bombings*. Atlanta, GA: Centers for Disease Control and Prevention; 2007. http://www.bt.cdc.gov/masscasualties/pdf/surgecapacity.pdf. Accessed June 30, 2009.

20. Auf der Heide E. Principles of hospital disaster planning. In: Hogan DE, Burstein JL. *Disaster Medicine*. Philadelphia, PA: Lippincott Williams and Wilkins; 2007.

21. Association for Professionals in Infection Control and Epidemiology Inc, Center for the Study of Bioterrorism and Emerging Infections. *Mass Casualty Disaster Plan Checklist: A Template for Healthcare Facilities*. http://bioterrorism.slu.edu/bt/quick/disasterplan.pdf. Accessed June 30, 2009.

22. *The Federal Response to Hurricane Katrina: Lessons Learned*. Washington, DC: The White House; 2006. http://georgewbush-whitehouse.archives.gov/reports/katrina-lessons-learned/. Accessed June 30, 2009.

23. Select Bipartisan Committee to Investigate the Preparation for and Response to Hurricane Katrina, U.S. House of Representatives. *A Failure of Initiative: The Final Report of the Select Bipartisan Committee to Investigate the Preparation for and Response to Hurricane Katrina*. Washington, DC: US House of Representatives; 2006. http://katrina.house.gov/. Accessed June 30, 2009.

24. Senate Committee on Homeland Security and Governmental Affairs. *Hurricane Katrina: A Nation Still Unprepared*. Washington, DC: US Senate; 2006. http://www.gpoaccess.gov/serialset/creports/katrinanation.html. Accessed June 30, 2009.

25. Centers for Disease Control and Prevention. *Crisis and Emergency Risk Communication*. Atlanta, GA: CDC; 2002. http://www.bt.cdc.gov/cerc/pdf/CERC-SEPT02.pdf. Accessed June 30, 2009.

26. Centers for Disease Control and Prevention. The Health Alert Network (HAN). http://www.bt.cdc.gov/DocumentsApp/HAN/han.asp. Accessed June 30, 2009.

CHAPTER FOUR

The Disaster Health System

4.1 PURPOSE

This chapter discusses the essential components of federal, state, regional, and community disaster health systems, including the role of the public and private health sectors.

4.2 LEARNING OBJECTIVES

After completing this chapter, readers should be able to:

➤ Describe key concepts and principles underlying the National Incident Management System.

➤ Given the all-hazards approach to disaster management, identify support services that need to be integrated into regional, community, and institutional emergency response systems.

➤ Describe the roles of various response entities (ie, in the public, private, and military sectors) in providing a coordinated response to a disaster or other public health emergency.

➤ Identify opportunities in the community for volunteering assistance in a disaster or other public health emergency.

4.3   DISASTER MEDICINE AND PUBLIC HEALTH PREPAREDNESS COMPETENCIES ADDRESSED

This chapter addresses the following competencies as delineated in Appendix E of this manual.

➤ Describe the purpose and relevance of the National Response Framework, National Incident Management System, Hospital Incident Command System, and Emergency Support Function 8 to regional, community, and institutional disaster response.

➤ Describe global, federal, regional, state, local, institutional, organizational, and private industry disaster support services, including the rationale for the integration and coordination of these systems.

4.4   OPENING VIGNETTE*

The worst terrorist attack on US soil occurred on September 11, 2001, at the World Trade Center in New York City. While most people are familiar with this event and its aftermath, it is a notable example of how a disaster health system responds to a large-scale event. Many local resources responded to this event, including public health, hospitals, emergency medical services (EMS), police, fire, and utilities, while continuing to provide their regular day-to-day services. There was a need for central coordination of all of these responding organizations, which was complicated by the fact that the emergency management command center at No. 7 World Trade Center also fell when the Twin Towers collapsed. After heavy losses were sustained by New York City Fire Department/ EMS and the New York Police Department, federal assistance was called upon. To enhance the response, the Stafford Act was invoked, which gave statutory authority to the Federal Emergency Management Agency (FEMA) to respond to the event and provide assistance to the city.** Unique to the World Trade Center disaster was the military and national security aspect as well as the combination of disasters: fire, water, smoke, biohazard potential, environmental hazards, and transportation. The 2001 World Trade Center disaster is an excellent case study of the interaction of federal and local government resources as well as private sector resources.

---

* Adapted from Landesman LY. *Public Health Management of Disasters: The Practice Guide.* Washington, DC: American Public Health Association; 2001.

** The Robert T. Stafford Disaster Relief and Emergency Assistance Act, PL 100–707, signed November 23, 1988, amended PL 93–288 of 1974 (42 USC 5121), which gives statutory authority to FEMA to carry out most federal disaster response activities.

4.5 INTRODUCTION

Response to a disaster event is not the responsibility of any single agency or group. The sheer size of these events and the numbers of people involved require cooperation among numerous agencies and individuals. This includes all levels of government and private sector responders. These agencies and responders come together to establish and implement a disaster health system. They must be "interoperable," or able to work together in their response to decrease duplication of effort, increase efficiency, and protect the safety of the community, as well as responders. A key means of improving the disaster health system response is leadership and management. This is achieved largely through use of the National Incident Management System (NIMS), which is discussed in this chapter in Section 4.7.2. Further, all potential responding and participating agencies must be aware of their roles before an event and understand how they fit into the larger disaster health system. It is also important for all individuals to realize that they play a role in disaster response as well, in terms of personal preparedness and the opportunity to support community disaster response through volunteerism.

4.6 COMPONENTS OF THE DISASTER HEALTH SYSTEM

4.6.1 Emergency Management System

Emergency management systems, which exist at the agency, local, state, and federal levels, ensure coordination of resources in the response to a disaster or public health emergency. Typically, emergency management is coordinated in emergency operations centers (EOCs), which are described in more detail in Chapter 6. These are physical locations where representatives from all the responding and collaborating agencies or departments within an agency go during an event to coordinate or integrate their responses. During a given incident there may be several levels of EOCs. For example, during a major industrial fire, the county where the event occurs may activate or "stand up" their EOC to coordinate the countywide response. Representatives from police, fire, EMS, local hospitals, local utilities, public health, etc, may be included. Meanwhile, the local trauma center may stand up its own EOC to coordinate the response within the trauma center itself; this would include representatives from the emergency department, patient/family relations, transport services, and others (in some medical institutions the terminology varies, and "command post" may be used.) The countywide EOC would have a health care representative who would communicate and coordinate activities by contacting the trauma center

EOC. Representatives at the trauma center EOC would then disseminate information and directions to their respective departments. In this way information will be quickly and accurately provided to all agencies as well as disseminated down to the individual provider level. If an event were very large, a state might initiate its own EOC and work with the local municipality EOC to coordinate all of their efforts. National standards for response management are promulgated by NIMS, which is discussed in Section 4.7.2.

An example of one emergency management system is the Boston Emergency Management Agency (BEMA).[1] In a disaster, BEMA activates its EOC, where representatives from all agencies gather. The EOC also coordinates events and serves as a liaison with the mayor's office and the Massachusetts State EOC.

BEMA houses the city's comprehensive emergency management plan, including all of its annexes, which is available for review by individuals or groups as necessary. The plan provides a chain of designated authorities to ensure that proper notifications are made and resources readied. There are special annexes for certain emergencies, eg, floods or bioterrorism. The plan generally has been implemented about once a year, usually during severe snowstorms. It is also drilled frequently in order to identify gaps and make amendments.

Nationally, the Centers for Disease Control and Prevention (CDC) EOC, which focuses largely on national responses to public health emergencies, natural disasters, and significant technolgical disasters, does not typically involve fire and police assets but may provide guidance to local and state EOCs in these areas. The CDC EOC is described in the box below. At an even higher level, the Secretary for Health and Human Services (HHS) has an EOC that is staffed 24 hours a day; it can be activated fully in response to incidents and disasters and coordinates with other federal departments and agencies.

The CDC EOC

The CDC EOC was established in 2003 to serve as CDC's command center for monitoring and coordinating CDC's emergency response to public health threats in the United States and abroad.

WHAT ARE THE FUNCTIONS OF THE CDC EOC?

The EOC allows CDC to maintain situational awareness of public health–related events at the international, national, state, and local levels. Staffed around the clock, it serves as CDC's central point of contact for reporting public health threats and supports the US Department of Health and Human Services (HHS) Secretary's Operations Center.

During an emergency response, the CDC EOC brings together scientists from across CDC to efficiently exchange information and connect with public health emergency response partners. For multistate or severe emergencies, CDC provides additional public health resources and coordinates response efforts across multiple jurisdictions, both domestically and abroad. The current 24,000-square-foot EOC facility became operational in 2006 and can accommodate up to 230 personnel per shift when fully staffed for two to three shifts per day to handle situations ranging from local interests to worldwide events. CDC's Division of Emergency Operations manages the EOC.

To support state and local efforts during an emergency response, EOC staff coordinates deployment of CDC staff and equipment that CDC responders may need. In addition, the EOC has the capability to transport life-supporting medications, samples/specimens, equipment, and personnel at any time anywhere in the world via aircraft that can be launched within 2 hours of notification for domestic and 6 hours for international responses.

4.6.2   The Public Health System

Overview.   Because it usually works behind the scenes, the public health system is often underappreciated and most citizens are unaware of its broad mission, which is to prevent disease and injuries. When the public health system succeeds, it is seldom recognized because it means a major event has been averted. During a mass casualty event, such as a widespread influenza outbreak or an act of terrorism, it is critical that the emergency care community and public health system work closely and efficiently to mitigate potential health impacts.

What Is Public Health?   *Public health* can be defined as a complex network of people, systems, and organizations that work together to ensure the conditions necessary to live healthy lives. The overarching mission of public health is to promote physical and mental health and prevent disease, injury, and disability.[2]

The public health system focuses on health and safety issues affecting *populations* rather than individual patients, the latter being the responsibility of the private health system. The public health system seeks to promote healthy behaviors, ensure the quality and accessibility of health services, and recognize emerging health threats that affect entire communities, states, or nations. In contrast, the private health system seeks to prevent, delay, and treat disease, injury, and disability, as well as promote healthier lifestyles, in *individual* patients. The public health system also serves as a "safety net" by linking people to needed personal health services and ensures the provision of health care when it is otherwise unavailable from the private sector in the community.

FIGURE 4-1
Ten essential services
provided by public health

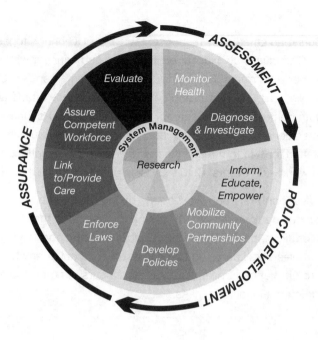

The fundamental obligations of public health agencies are to (1) prevent epidemics and the spread of disease; (2) protect against environmental hazards; (3) prevent injuries; (4) promote and encourage healthy behaviors and mental health; (5) respond to disasters and assist communities in recovery; and (6) ensure the quality and accessibility of health services.[2,3] In service of these fundamental obligations, public health provides 10 essential services, depicted in Figure 4-1.

Essential Public Health Services

➤ Monitor health status to identify community health problems

➤ Diagnose and investigate health problems and health hazards in the community

➤ Inform, educate, and empower people about health issues

➤ Mobilize community partnerships to identify and solve health problems

➤ Develop policies and plans that support individual and community health efforts

➤ Enforce laws and regulations that protect health and ensure safety

➤ Link people to needed personal health services and assure the provision of health care when otherwise unavailable

➤ Assure a competent public health and personal health care workforce

➤ Evaluate effectiveness, accessibility, and quality of personal and population-based health services

➤ Research for new insights and innovative solutions to health problems

Public Health Infrastructure. Early detection and control of a public health emergency depends on a strong and flexible public health system at the local, state, and federal levels and on the vigilance of health workers, who may be the first to observe and report unusual illnesses or injuries. The public health infrastructure protects the nation against the spread of disease and environmental and occupational hazards. It is composed of three interrelated components: a competent workforce, robust information systems, and strong organizational capacities.[4]

Integration of public health and the emergency care community—first responders, EMS, hospital emergency departments, trauma centers, volunteers, and so on—is critical to successful disaster response. Examples of communities in which strong linkages exist have been documented by the CDC's Terrorist Injuries: Information, Dissemination, and Exchange project.[5]

Public Health Case Study

In January 1992, dozens of previously healthy individuals from the state of Washington began streaming into physician offices with similar complaints, including nausea, vomiting, and diarrhea.[6] Alarmed by the unusual nature and number of patients presenting to his office, one physician called the local health department to raise concern. Public health investigators moved into action by calling hospitals and physicians in the vicinity to determine whether they were seeing patients with similar symptoms. Health officials interviewed all sick patients with similar symptoms to determine whether they shared any common exposure.

This detective work quickly identified that more than 90% of sick persons had eaten at a local chain restaurant within the last 10 days. Stool specimens from all sick patients revealed the same bacterium, *Escherichia coli* O157:H7. Uncooked hamburger meat from the implicated restaurant also contained the same strain of *E coli* O157:H7 with an identical DNA fingerprint.

Armed with this information, public health authorities activated a risk communication plan and control strategy by immediately informing the public about the infection and its source, and warning them not to eat uncooked or undercooked hamburger. Furthermore, 250,000 potentially contaminated hamburgers were recalled and removed from stores and restaurants and destroyed.

Overall, 501 patients were identified, including 151 who were hospitalized; 45 patients developed renal failure, and 3 died. Through early detection and rapid response, an estimated 800 additional cases were prevented. And it all started by one call from a concerned physician to his local health department.

FIGURE 4-2
The six basic types of
EMS services

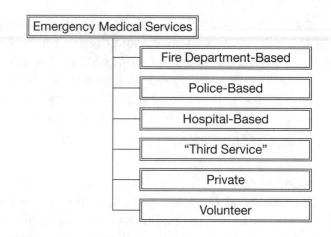

4.6.3   EMS Systems

People's lives often depend on the quick reaction and competent care of EMS. Incidents as varied as automobile crashes, heart attacks, falls, childbirth, and gunshot wounds all require immediate medical attention. EMS responder provide this vital service as they care for and transport the sick or injured to a medical facility. EMS systems vary widely in organizational type. There are six basic types of EMS services (Figure 4-2): (1) fire department–based; (2) police-based; (3) hospital-based; (4) "third service," eg, services organized under a public health department; (5) private; and (6) volunteer.[7] The type of EMS services varies greatly from community to community; typically, no one organizational type provides all of the care in any one state, and often in any one city.

Specialized EMS services also exist, such as helicopter response and transport teams. Most EMS agencies have medical directors who provide real-time medical advice as well as written protocols to guide patient treatment.

EMS providers also vary in type. The National Registry of Emergency Medical Technicians certifies emergency medical service providers, reflecting their level of qualification and training, on five levels: first responder; EMT-basic; EMT-intermediate, which has two levels called 1985 and 1999; and paramedic.[8] Some states, however, have their own certification programs and use distinct names and titles.

EMT-basic represents the first component of the emergency medical technician (EMT) system. An EMT trained at this level is prepared to care for patients at the scene of an injury and while transporting patients by ambulance to the hospital. The EMT-basic has the emergency skills to assess a patient's condition and manage respiratory, cardiac, and trauma emergencies.

The EMT-intermediate has more advanced training. The specific tasks that those certified at this level are allowed to perform vary greatly from state to state but generally include establishing intravenous access and providing advanced airway procedures.

EMT-paramedics provide the most extensive prehospital care. In addition to carrying out the procedures of the other levels, paramedics may administer medications, interpret electrocardiograms, and use monitors and other complex equipment. However, as with EMT-intermediate, what paramedics are permitted to do varies by state.

In an emergency, EMTs and paramedics are typically dispatched by a 911 operator to the scene, where they often work with police and firefighters. Once they arrive, EMTs and paramedics assess the nature of the patient's condition while trying to determine whether the patient has any preexisting medical conditions. Following medical protocols and guidelines, they provide appropriate emergency care and transport the patient, often communicating from the field with the receiving agency. At the medical facility, EMTs and paramedics help transfer patients to the emergency department and report their observations and actions to emergency department staff. After each run, EMTs and paramedics replace used supplies and check equipment. They may also need to decontaminate the interior of the ambulance, depending on the nature of the patient's illness or injury.

4.6.4 Private Sector Health Care (Trauma Care System, Acute Health Care, Chronic Care, and Rehabilitation Systems)

The private health care system generally seeks to prevent, delay, and treat disease, injury, and disability, as well as promote healthier lifestyles in individual patients. There are many types of facilities that address individual needs along the continuum of care, from acute needs to chronic long-term care. While hospitals and primary care providers are able to provide acute care for most noncritical patients, trauma centers are medically sophisticated facilities that are appropriately staffed to treat the more seriously injured patients. Trauma centers are hospitals that have been designated by either their state or the American College of Surgeons on the basis of capabilities and staffing. In a small event such as an explosion due to a gas leak with several victims at a single house, a trauma center will likely have sufficient resources to meet the needs of all the victims. However, as an event increases in size and scope, eg, an explosion in a multiunit apartment building, the number of needed health care resoruces will increase. This may include using non–acute care facilities to provide acute care or moving patients prematurely from acute care facilities to other types of facilities so there is sufficient capacity to meet the needs of the event. However, all of these scenarios need to be planned in advance and well coordinated in order to comprise an effective community trauma system.

In most states, there is an organized trauma care system designed to deliver the full spectrum of care to injured patients within a defined geographic area, starting at the time of injury, through transport to an acute care facility, to rehabilitative care. The system represents *dual-use capacity*—the system is designed to

FIGURE 4-3
Trauma care system operations

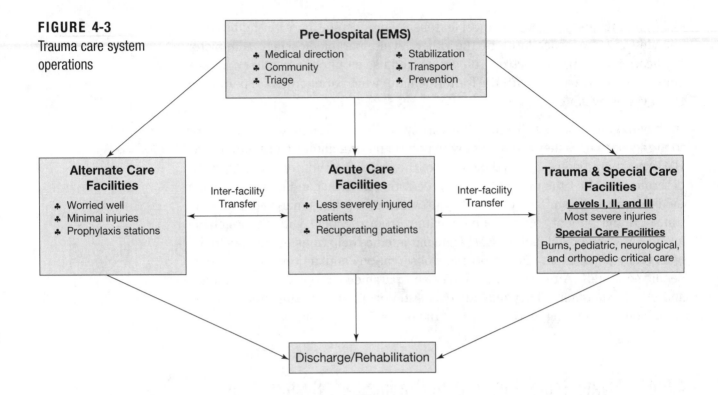

provide ongoing trauma care at all levels, as well as being ready to ramp up to meet disaster conditions, thereby helping to organize the disaster response.[9]

The day-to-day operational aspects of the trauma care system are depicted in Figure 4-3.[10] The discussion and graphics apply primarily to adult trauma centers. However, it must be noted that there are also specialty care facilities for neonatal care, pediatric patients, burn patients, and orthopedic or neurologic critical care.

Trauma centers, representing the acute care capacity of the system, are designed with scalability in mind, both systemwide and within each individual trauma center. One fundamental tenet of the trauma center is its integrated, multidisciplinary approach to care. In most trauma centers—especially level I and II centers—the "normal" cadre of medical personnel, including trauma surgeons, emergency medicine physicians, and emergency department nurses, is frequently augmented by the addition of anesthesiologists, radiologists, internal medicine physicians, infectious disease specialists, obstetrician-gynecologists, cardiologists, neurologists and neurosurgeons, pulmonary specialists, toxicologists, specialty nurses, and many others.

The American College of Surgeons guidelines classify trauma centers into four levels: I, II, III, and IV.[11]

Level I: A regional tertiary care facility with designated trauma care facilities that serves large cities or densely populated areas and is capable of treating the most severely injured patients. Level I trauma centers must have immediate availability of trauma surgeons, specialized surgeons (eg, neurosurgeons and orthopedic surgeons), physician specialists, anesthesiologists, specialized nurses, resuscitative equipment, and surgical facilities. Level I trauma centers also conduct research and injury prevention activities.

Level II: Similar to level I but without research and prevention activity requirements. A level II trauma center may be located in densely populated areas close to a level I trauma center, in which case its function is to work cooperatively with the level I center to optimize treatment resources for seriously injured people in their area. Level II centers may also be located in less densely populated areas and serve as the lead trauma facility for that geographic area.

Level III: A facility that provides assessment, resuscitation, and emergency surgery and, if indicated, transfers patients to a level I or II trauma center. Level III centers often serve communities that do not have a level I or II trauma center.

Level IV: A hospital or clinic in a remote area designed to resuscitate and stabilize patients and arrange for their transfer to the closest appropriate level of trauma care.

Even in areas replete with several trauma centers, other acute care facilities play an important role in disaster response. They can be called on to provide acute care to less critically injured patients, or act as staging areas for triage of patients to other facilities. Rehabilitation centers can also be used as "overflow" facilities for noncritically injured patients transferred from trauma centers to provide more capacity within the trauma center itself.

Alternative care sites can be used in a disaster to care for "overflow" patients transferred from large hospitals and trauma centers to make room in these facilities for more acutely injured people. Such sites may include rehabilitation hospitals, nursing homes, and community health centers. Alternate care sites are most effective when they are identified and planned for in advance to ensure the capability and resources to care for patients.

4.6.5   Businesses, Corporations, and Nongovernmental Organizations (NGOs)[12]

While it may not seem intuitive that businesses and corporations would play a role in disaster response, it is important to remember that a disaster event can affect a number of systems and services that are integral to public health and safety. For example, a major explosion or fire may disrupt the services of local utilities, which could lead to persons with special needs requiring assistance because their assistive devices, such as home ventilators, will not operate. Even individuals without special needs may be affected if utilities are interrupted for long periods of time. For example, during a major ice storm that resulted in extended power outages, individuals and families had to be reminded to dispose of food that might have been defrosted and then refrozen when the utilities were restored, to reduce the risk of foodborne illness. Further, there may be scene hazards such as downed power lines that only utility companies can address.

These issues may seem obvious, but there are also responder needs, such as their own personal health and safety as well as knowing that their families and personal assets are safe, as discussed in Chapter 2. These issues are likely to be too broad for the individual responder's agency to provide. For example, in a major infectious disease outbreak, schools and other child care providers may close to reduce the spread of the disease. However, this may have the unintended consequence of preventing or delaying health providers with children in reporting for duty because they have no one to look after their children. Further, the basic needs of responders and those affected by the event must be provided for, such as food, sanitation, clothing, and safe places to rest. Without the involvement of NGOs and private businesses, these needs may not be met and will reduce the ability of agencies to respond. An entire community's recovery from an event will be slowed if these services cannot be provided. It is important that NGOs and businesses be involved in community disaster planning so that these potential issues can be planned for and addressed before an event occurs.

Some NGOs are officially designated as support elements to national response capabilities. According to the National Response Framework, the *American Red Cross* is a supporting agency to the mass care functions of emergency support function (ESF) 6 (see the discussion of ESFs later in this chapter). It does not direct other NGOs, but the American Red Cross takes the lead in the integration of efforts of the national NGOs that provide mass care services during response operations. Also, the National Voluntary Organizations Active in Disaster (NVOAD) is the forum in which organizations share knowledge and resources throughout the disaster cycle (preparation, response, and recovery) to help disaster survivors and their communities. This consortium of approximately 50 national organizations and 55 state and territory equivalents sends representatives to the Department of Homeland Security (DHS) and FEMA's national response coordination center to represent the voluntary organizations and assist in response coordination.

4.6.6   Community Groups and Citizen Volunteers

Depending on the size and scale of the disaster, private citizen volunteers may be called on to assist in the response. Many states are creating a registry of private physician and nurse volunteers to ask for assistance.

The Community Emergency Response Team (CERT) concept was developed and implemented by the Los Angeles City Fire Department in 1985. It has grown into a national program designed to educate the public about disaster preparedness for hazards that may impact their area and to train them in basic disaster response skills, such as fire safety, light search and rescue, team organization, and disaster medical operations.[13] CERT members are able to assist others in their neighborhood or workplace after an event when professional responders are not immediately available. They also provide useful information to responders when they do arrive and support the responders' efforts as directed. More than 1100 communities currently have CERT programs, with training sponsored by emergency management agencies, fire departments, and police departments.

Another organized volunteer response is the Medical Reserve Corps (MRC). The MRC consists of groups of specially trained volunteers whose goal is to improve the health and safety of communities across the country by organizing and utilizing public health, medical, and other volunteers. Currently, there are more than 850 MRC units across the country utilizing the services of more than 189,000 volunteers.[14]

MRC units are community based and function as a means to locally organize and utilize volunteers who want to donate their time and expertise to prepare for and respond to emergencies and promote healthy living throughout the year. MRC volunteers supplement existing emergency and public health resources.

MRC volunteers include medical and public health professionals such as physicians, nurses, mental health providers, pharmacists, dentists, veterinarians, and epidemiologists. Additionally, other community members—interpreters, chaplains, office workers, legal advisors, and others—also fill key support positions.

MRC volunteers may support communities in need nationwide. When the southeast was battered by hurricanes in 2004, MRC volunteers in the affected areas helped communities by filling in at local hospitals, assisting their neighbors at local shelters, and providing first aid to those injured by the storms. During this 2-month period, more than 30 MRC units worked as part of the relief efforts, including those whose volunteers were called in from across the country to assist the American Red Cross and FEMA.

During the 2005 hurricane season, MRC members provided support for American Red Cross health services, mental health, and shelter operations. MRC members also supported the HHS response and recovery efforts by staffing special needs shelters and community health centers and health clinics, and assisting health assessment teams in the Gulf Coast region. More than 1,500 MRC members deployed outside of their local jurisdiction. Of these, almost 200 volunteers from 25 MRC units were activated by HHS, and more than 400 volunteers from more than 80 local MRC units were activated to support American Red Cross disaster operations in Gulf Coast areas.

MRCs fall under the jurisdiction of the Office of the Civilian Volunteer Medical Reserve Corps (OCVMRC), which is housed within the Office of the US Surgeon General. The OCVMRC functions as a clearinghouse for information and best practices to help communities establish, implement, and maintain MRC units nationwide. The OCVMRC sponsors an annual leadership conference, hosts a Web site, and coordinates with local, state, regional, and national organizations and agencies to help communities achieve their local visions for public health and emergency preparedness. Including local MRC units in planning, training, and exercises among regional partners builds depth to a community's response force.

The American Red Cross organizes local chapters that may also assist in a disaster. Specifically, the Red Cross is involved in ESF 6, Mass Care, Housing, and Human Services (described later in this chapter), and frequently takes the lead in training and supervising their volunteers, setting up shelters, feeding and clothing affected individuals and families, and tracking the location of displaced persons.

These organized activities are important because, during an event, many people will want to assist in the response. However, allowing unknown volunteers access to disaster scenes may have safety implications. There may not be a way to verify volunteer credentials to ensure that they are not actually intent on doing harm (eg, part of a terrorist plot) or to ensure they are qualified to engage in the type of service they are offering to provide (eg, nonlicensed providers posing as physicians). Further, there have been incidents in which off-duty personnel responded to disaster scenes and were killed because they entered unsecured areas without proper safety equipment. This not only affects the volunteer and his or her family but also expands the work of responders by creating additional victims at the event. Credentialing programs that verify licensing and skill levels in order to prevent such incidents have been developed at the state and local levels.

4.6.7 The Media

The media play several important roles in disaster response. First, they inform disaster managers about the size and scope of the disaster, many times before public safety, public health, and medical personnel are able to assess the situation themselves. They have resources that enable them to get to the scene quickly, record the sequelae of the disaster, and report it in real time. Many emergency managers have mentioned how heavily they rely on news stations such as CNN.

Another critical role is that of risk communication to the general public. The National Academy of Sciences defines *risk communication* as "an interactive process of exchange of information and opinion among individuals, groups, and institutions. It involves multiple messages about the nature of risk and other messages, not strictly about risk, that express concerns, opinions, or reactions to risk messages or to legal and institutional arrangements for risk management."[15]

Effectively communicating information during public health emergencies remains a significant challenge. Such communication needs to be carefully planned and implemented, and it must be properly integrated with emergency management operations. Emergencies present a unique challenge to the internal media-relations capabilities of health agencies; therefore, preparation and development of trusted relationships—*before* an event occurs—is vital. It is all too easy to be caught unprepared, especially for short-notice or demanding media interviews. Conversely, well-constructed and properly delivered media messages can inform and calm a worried public, reduce misinformation, and focus attention on what is most important. These messages must be delivered by a credible and trusted spokesperson from the responders as well as from the media itself. Poor communication can lead to the perception that the agency is incompetent, uncaring, or dishonest. Proper communication will reach more people with a clear and credible public health message. Effective media communication is therefore a key responsibility of public health, public safety, and emergency care community professionals who are designated as information officers during emergencies. Agency spokespersons who will be addressing the media and/or the public should be credible, authoritative, and well informed.

4.6.8   The Military and Veterans Affairs System

The federal response to a disaster may include directing the National Guard and the resources of the Department of Defense (DOD) to assist in evacuation, and Veterans Affairs (VA) hospitals to absorb patient overload. The National Guard is activated by the governor of the state and is not formally a DOD asset. Reserve military units may be activated for disaster response and support by DOD along with tasking of active units, depending on the circumstances of the disaster and other requirements. For these assets to be used reliably, they must be integrated into the local response with good lines of communication.

4.6.9   Public Safety Systems

Safety is a key aspect of the DISASTER Paradigm™ in terms of safety and security (*S*) and assessing for hazards (*A*). As such, public safety is a key aspect of the disaster health system beyond the assistance that public safety responders can provide for health care. First and foremost, public safety agencies are responsible for maintaining scene safety and security. For example, it is important that routes to and from the scene of the event are clear so that assets may be brought to the scene and patients may be delivered to definitive care facilities. Further, by restricting scene access, the risk of secondary attacks on responders may be mitigated and the number of self-deployed volunteers on the scene will be reduced.

While all responders should assess the scene for hazards before entering the area, only specially trained public safety personal may be able to identify certain scene hazards such as secondary devices or chemical hazards that are stored at or near the scene. Assessing the scene for hazards may require the cooperation of many local agencies, including law enforcement, fire protection, hazardous materials (HAZMAT), and bomb teams. For example, during a fire at a local manufacturing plant, fire officials might need to contact local health officials to obtain a list of chemicals that are stored at the site. Additional experts and HAZMAT personnel might need to be contacted to determine what risk those chemicals pose given the circumstances of the event. Community planning and preparation well in advance of an event would identify hazardous materials or circumstances for various businesses and expedite the most effective response to the event.

Other public safety functions might include decontamination and search and rescue. In the event that decontamination is required, special care must be taken not to contaminate and compromsie critical response assets such as ambulances or local hospitals.

4.6.10   Mortuary Care Services

Caring for the dead is an important part of disaster response because it has implications for criminal investigations, public health, and recovery. Deceased victims at a disaster event should be moved as little as possible to preserve evidence so that the perpetrators of an event can be brought to justice. The chain of evidence must be preserved, so the deceased's belongings and any fragmented body parts should be kept with the deceased; there should be proper documentation by date, time, and initials of each person who has had possession of any articles or the body. These practices will also aid in victim identification. Further, decomposing bodies can create public health risks, particularly if they are contaminated with chemical or biologic agents. Therefore, it is critical that plans be developed for proper storage and handling of deceased victims. This is further complicated by the fact that the handling of these remains may have implications for a community's recovery, including the emotional needs of family and friends and long-term implications for locations that are selected for storage.

Depending on the location of the incident and the number of casualties, the care of the dead may be led by a Disaster Mortuary Response Team (DMORT), sometimes assisted by other on-site physicians. DMORTs generally include 25 primary responders and a team of up to 100 additional members. Teams include funeral directors, law enforcement agents, firefighters, fingerprint experts, photographers, pathologists, medical examiners, radiologists, mental health staff, and support personnel. In the United States there are 10 teams, one for each FEMA district.

All responders involved in the care of the dead must have a basic understanding of the principles that guide this work:

➤ The first priority is the safety of the responders.

➤ The second priority is the removal of bodies from the scene. Responders should keep deceased individuals' personal belongings with them to assist in their identification.

➤ Because the site of a terrorist attack is a crime scene, responders must preserve the chain of custody of evidence when removing personal effects and other materials found with and around victims. Chain of custody is knowing where each article and body is at all times, with proper documentation by date, time, and initials of each person who has had possession of that article or body.

When it is not feasible or possible to transport dead bodies to a morgue, responders should set up a temporary field morgue. Bodies should be refrigerated as soon as possible at 2° to 4°C (35° to 40°F). Refrigerated trucks, ice rinks, or other refrigerated facilities can be used for this purpose. Until bodies can be refrigerated, they should be kept in a cool area. When refrigeration is not possible, mass burial may be necessary to prevent disease.

4.7 ROLE OF THE FEDERAL GOVERNMENT IN DISASTER RESPONSE

4.7.1 National Preparedness Guidelines and Directives

National preparedness guidelines grew largely out of the attacks on September 11, 2001. The creation of DHS brought with it several Presidential directives and a concomitant rethinking of disaster preparedness and response. Two key directives were the development of the National Incident Management System (NIMS), guidelines for organizing a coordinated, coherent response to disasters; and the National Response Framework (NRF), a more specific guide to how the nation conducts all-hazards response built on scalable, flexible, and adaptable coordinating structures to align key roles and responsibilities across the nation. While these are described in detail in the following sections, Homeland Security Presidential Directive (HSPD-21), released in October 2007, established a national strategy for public health and medical preparedness that builds on the principles articulated in *Biodefense for the 21st Century* (April 2004) to protect the American public by utilizing an all-hazards approach to disaster preparedness, education, training, and response.[16]

4.7.2 The National Incident Management System (NIMS)

Incidents, ranging from natural disasters to explosions, typically begin and end locally and are managed on a daily basis at the lowest possible geographic, organizational, and jurisdictional level. However, there are instances in which successful incident management operations depend on the involvement of multiple jurisdictions, levels of government, functional agencies, and/or emergency responder disciplines. These instances require effective and efficient coordination across this broad spectrum of organizations and activities.

> **The National Incident Management System (NIMS)**
>
> The NIMS provides a nationwide template enabling federal, state, local, and tribal governments and the private sector and NGOs to work together effectively and efficiently to prevent, prepare for, respond to, and recover from domestic incidents regardless of cause, size, or complexity.

In recognition of this, on February 28, 2003, the President issued HSPD-5, Management of Domestic Incidents, which directed the Secretary of Homeland Security to develop and administer a National Incident Management System.[17] This system provides a consistent nationwide template to enable federal, state, tribal, and local governments, NGOs, and the private sector to work together to prevent, protect against, respond to, recover from, and mitigate the effects of incidents, regardless of cause, size, location, or complexity. This consistency provides the foundation for utilization of NIMS for all incidents, ranging from daily occurrences to incidents requiring a coordinated federal response.

NIMS uses a systematic approach to integrate the best existing processes and methods into a unified national framework for incident management. *Incident management* refers to how incidents are managed across all Homeland Security activities, including prevention, protection, response, mitigation, and recovery.

This framework forms the basis for interoperability and compatibility that will, in turn, enable a diverse set of public and private organizations to conduct well-integrated and effective emergency management and incident response operations. *Emergency management* is the coordination and integration of all activities necessary to build, sustain, and improve the capability to prepare for, protect against, respond to, recover from, or mitigate against threatened or actual natural disasters, acts of terrorism, or other human-caused disasters. It does this through a core set of concepts, principles, procedures, organizational processes, terminology, and standard requirements applicable to a broad community of NIMS users.

NIMS is *not* an operational incident management or resource allocation plan. It represents a core set of doctrines, concepts, principles, terminology, and organizational processes that enables effective, efficient, and collaborative incident management. NIMS is based on the premise that utilization of a common incident management framework will give emergency management/ response personnel a flexible but standardized system for emergency management and incident response activities. NIMS is flexible because the system components can be used to develop plans, processes, procedures, agreements, and roles for all types of incidents; it is scalable to any incident regardless of cause, size, location, or complexity. Additionally, NIMS provides an organized set of standardized operational structures, which is critical in allowing disparate organizations and agencies to work together in a predictable, coordinated manner.

HSPD-5 also required the Secretary of Homeland Security to develop the National Response Plan, which has been superseded by the National Response Framework (NRF), discussed in greater detail below. The NRF is a guide to how the nation conducts all-hazards response. The NRF identifies the key principles, as well as the roles and structures that organize national response. Further, it describes special circumstances in which the federal government exercises a larger role, including incidents in which federal interests are involved and catastrophic incidents in which a state would require significant support.

HSPD-5 requires all federal departments and agencies to adopt NIMS and to use it in their individual incident management programs and activities, as well as in support of all actions taken to assist state, tribal, and local governments. The directive requires federal departments and agencies to make adoption of NIMS by state, tribal, and local organizations a condition for federal preparedness assistance (through grants, contracts, and other activities). NIMS recognizes the role that NGOs and the private sector have in preparedness and activities to prevent, protect against, respond to, recover from, and mitigate the effects of incidents.

Building on the foundation provided by existing emergency management and incident response systems used by jurisdictions, organizations, and functional disciplines at all levels, NIMS integrates best practices into a comprehensive framework for use nationwide by emergency management/response personnel in an all-hazards context. (Emergency management and response personnel include federal, state, territorial, tribal, substate, regional, and local governments, NGOs, private sector organizations, critical infrastructure owners and operators, and all other organizations and individuals who assume an emergency management role.) These best practices lay the groundwork for the components of NIMS and provide the mechanisms for the further development and refinement of supporting national standards, guidelines, protocols, systems, and technologies. NIMS fosters the development of specialized technologies that facilitate emergency management and incident response activities, and allows for the adoption of new approaches that will enable continuous refinement of the system over time. NIMS "training" is directed toward key personnel across all agencies in order to provide a mutual understanding of the concepts and create depth.

The Secretary of Homeland Security, through the National Integration Center, Incident Management Systems Integration Division (formerly known as the NIMS Integration Center), publishes the standards, guidelines, and compliance protocols for determining whether a federal, state, tribal, or local government has implemented NIMS.

4.7.3 National Response Framework (NRF)

The NRF is a guide to how the nation conducts all-hazards response. It is built on scalable, flexible, and adaptable coordinating structures to align key roles and responsibilities across the nation. It describes specific authorities and best practices for managing incidents that range from the serious, but purely local, to large-scale terrorist attacks or catastrophic natural disasters. Importantly, the NRF builds on NIMS, which provides a consistent template for managing incidents. In this context, the term *response* includes immediate actions to save lives, protect property and the environment, and meet basic human needs. *Response* also includes the execution of emergency plans and actions to support short-term recovery.

The NRF, based on the principles of NIMS, is an all-hazards plan that provides the structure and mechanisms for a national policy and operational coordination for domestic incident management. Consistent with the model provided in the NIMS, the NRF can be partially or fully implemented in the context of a threat, anticipation of a significant event, or the response to a significant event. Selective implementation through the activation of one or more of the system's components allows maximum flexibility in meeting the unique operational and information-sharing requirements of the situation at hand and enabling effective interaction between various federal and nonfederal entities.[12]

4.7.4   Emergency Support Functions

Federal response consists of 15 areas, or ESFs. The ESFs provide the structure for coordinating federal interagency support for incidents of national significance. The ESF structure includes mechanisms used to provide federal support to states and federal-to-federal support, both for declared disasters and emergencies under the Stafford Act and for non–Stafford Act incidents as defined in HSPD-5.

The ESF structure provides mechanisms for interagency coordination during all phases of incident management. Some departments and agencies provide resources for response, support, and program implementation during the early stage of an event, while others are more prominent in the recovery phase.

The 15 ESFs are as follows:

ESF 1:   Transportation

ESF 2:   Communication

ESF 3:   Public Works and Engineering

ESF 4:   Firefighting

ESF 5:   Emergency Management

ESF 6:   Mass Care, Housing, and Human Services

ESF 7:   Resource Support

ESF 8:   *Public Health and Medical Services*

ESF 9:   Urban Search and Rescue

ESF 10: Oil and Hazardous Materials Response

ESF 11: Agriculture and Natural Resources

ESF 12: Energy

ESF 13: Public Safety and Security

ESF 14: Long-term Community Recovery and Mitigation

ESF 15: External Affairs

The purpose of ESF 8, Public Health and Medical Services, is to provide US government assistance to supplement state and local responses in responding to public health and medical care needs after a disaster or a public health emergency, such as a pandemic. These resources are provided when state and local assets are overwhelmed and federal assistance has been requested.[18]

ESF 8 provides the mechanism for coordinated federal assistance to supplement state and local resources in response to public health and medical care needs for potential or actual incidents of national significance and/or during a developing potential health and medical emergency. ESF 8 is coordinated by the Secretary of HHS principally through the Assistant Secretary for Public Health Emergency Preparedness. ESF 8 resources can be activated through the Stafford Act or the Public Health Service Act (pending the availability of funds).

ESF 8 assists state and local governments in identifying and meeting the public health and medical needs of victims of an incident of national significance. This support is categorized in the following 18 functional areas:

Assessment of Health and Medical Needs. HHS, in collaboration with DHS, mobilizes and deploys ESF 8 personnel to support the Advance Emergency Response Team to assess public health and medical needs. This function includes assessment of the public health system/facility infrastructure.

Health Surveillance. HHS, in coordination with state health agencies, enhances existing surveillance systems to monitor the health of the general population and special high-risk populations, carry out field studies and investigations, monitor injury and disease patterns and potential disease outbreaks, and provide technical assistance and consultations on disease and injury prevention and precautions.

Medical Care Personnel. Immediate medical response capabilities are provided by assets internal to HHS, eg, US Public Health Service (USPHS) Commissioned Corps, and from ESF 8–supporting organizations, eg, the National Disaster Medical System (NDMS), which is currently housed within the Office of Preparedness and Emergency Operations, a division of HHS. The USPHS Rapid Deployment Forces (RDFs) were created in 2006 as part of the NRF's ESF 8 public health and medical asset provisions.[19] There are five RDFs, each with a workforce of more than 125 trained USPHS commissioned officers, although each RDF is scalable to provide only the resources needed. The Secretary and Assistant Secretary for Health have the authority to activate an RDF in response to requests made through the Surgeon General. The NDMS is discussed in Section 4.7.5.

The DOD may be requested to provide support in casualty clearing/staging and other missions as needed, although DOD is primarily involved in support for evacuation of patients or transportation under ESF 1. Further, HHS may seek individual clinical health and medical care specialists from the VA to assist state and local personnel.

Health, Medical, and Veterinary Equipment and Supplies.   In addition to deploying assets from the Strategic National Stockpile (SNS), described in Section 4.7.7, HHS may request DHS, DOD, or the VA to provide medical equipment and supplies, including medical, diagnostic, and radiation-emitting devices, pharmaceuticals, and biologic products in support of immediate medical response operations and for restocking health facilities in an area affected by a major disaster or emergency.

Patient Evacuation.   At the request of HHS, DOD coordinates with ESF 1, Transportation, to provide support for the evacuation of seriously ill or injured patients to locations where hospital care or outpatient services are available.

DOD is responsible for regulating and tracking patients transported on DOD assets to appropriate treatment facilities, eg, NDMS nonfederal hospitals.

Patient Care.   HHS may use its own resources and the Medical Reserve Corps, and request the VA, DOD, and DHS to provide available personnel to support inpatient hospital care and outpatient services to victims who become seriously ill or injured, regardless of location, which may include mass care shelters.

Food, Drug, Biologic, and Medical Device Safety.   HHS may work to ensure the safety and efficacy, and advise on the security, of regulated human and veterinary drugs, biologics (including blood and vaccines), medical devices (including radiation-emitting and screening devices), and other HHS-regulated products.

Blood, Organs, and Blood Products.   HHS monitors blood availability and maintains contact with the American Association of Blood Banks Interorganizational Task Force on Domestic Disasters and Acts of Terrorism and, as necessary, its individual members, to determine (1) the need for blood, blood products, and the supplies used in their manufacture, testing, and storage; (2) the ability of existing supply chain resources to meet these needs; and (3) any emergency measures needed to augment or replenish existing supplies.

Food Safety and Security.   HHS, in cooperation with ESF 11, Agriculture and Natural Resources, may use its resources to ensure the safety and security of federally regulated foods. (Note: HHS, through the Food and Drug Administration, has statutory authority for all domestic and imported food except meat, poultry, and egg products, which are under the authority of the US Department of Agriculture/Food Safety and Inspection Service.)

Agriculture Safety and Security.   HHS, in coordination with ESF 11, may work to ensure the safety and security of food-producing animals, animal feed, and therapeutics. (Note: HHS, through the Food and Drug Administration, has statutory authority for animal feed and for the approval of animal drugs intended for both therapeutic and nontherapeutic use in food animals as well as companion animals.)

Worker Safety and Health.   Under agreement with the US Department of Labor, that department is the lead federal agency for worker safety and health. ESF 8/HHS is a supporting agency.

All-Hazard Public Health and Medical Consultation, Technical Assistance, and Support.   ESF 8 may task HHS components and regional offices and request assistance from other ESF 8 partner organizations in assessing public health, medical, and veterinary medical effects resulting from all hazards. Such tasks may include assessing exposures on the general population and on high-risk population groups; conducting field investigations, including collection and analysis of relevant samples; providing advice on protective actions related to direct human and animal exposures, and on indirect exposure through contaminated food, drugs, water supply, and other media; and providing technical assistance and consultation on medical treatment, screening, and decontamination of injured or contaminated individuals. While state, tribal, and local officials retain primary responsibility for victim screening and decontamination operations, ESF 8 can deploy the National Medical Response Teams to assist with victim decontamination.

Behavioral Health Care.   ESF 8 may task HHS components and request assistance from other ESF 8 partner organizations in assessing mental health and substance abuse needs, including emotional, psychological, psychological first aid, behavioral, or cognitive limitations requiring assistance or supervision; providing disaster mental health training materials for workers; providing liaison with assessment, training, and program development activities undertaken by federal, state, tribal, or local mental health and substance abuse officials; and providing additional consultation as needed.

Public Health and Medical Information.   ESF 8 provides public health, disease, and injury prevention information that can be transmitted to members of the general public who are located in or near areas affected in languages and formats that are understandable to individuals with limited English proficiency and individuals with disabilities.

Vector Control.   ESF 8 may task HHS components and request assistance from other ESF 8 partner organizations, as appropriate, in assessing the threat of vector-borne diseases; conducting field investigations, including the collection and laboratory analysis of relevant samples; providing vector control equipment and supplies; providing technical assistance and consultation on protective actions regarding vector-borne diseases; and providing technical assistance and consultation on medical treatment of victims of vector-borne diseases.

Public Health Aspects of Potable Water/Wastewater and Solid Waste. ESF 8 may task HHS components and request assistance from other ESF 8 organizations to assist in assessing potable water, wastewater, solid waste disposal, and other environmental health issues related to public health in establishments holding, preparing, and/or serving food, drugs, or medical devices at retail and medical facilities, as well as examining and responding to public health effects from contaminated water; conducting field investigations, including collection and laboratory analysis of relevant samples; providing equipment and supplies as needed; and providing technical assistance and consultation.

Mass Fatality Management. ESF 8, when requested by state, tribal, or local officials, in coordination with its partner organizations, will assist the jurisdictional medicolegal authority and law enforcement agencies in the tracking and documenting of human remains and associated personal effects; reducing the hazard presented by chemically, biologically, or radiologically contaminated human remains (when indicated and possible); establishing temporary morgue facilities; determining the cause and manner of death; collecting antemortem data in a compassionate and culturally competent fashion from authorized individuals; performing postmortem data collection and documentation; identifying human remains by scientific means (eg, dental, pathology, anthropology, fingerprints, and, as indicated, DNA samples); preparing, processing, and returning human remains and personal effects to the authorized person(s) when possible; and providing technical assistance and consultation on fatality management and mortuary affairs. In the event that caskets are displaced, ESF 8 assists in identifying the human remains, replacing them in caskets, and reburying them in public cemeteries.

ESF 8 may task HHS components and request assistance from other ESF 8 partner organizations, as appropriate, to provide support to families of victims during the victim identification mortuary process.

Veterinary Medical Support.   ESF 8 will provide veterinary assistance to ESF 11. Support will include the amelioration of zoonotic disease and caring for research animals where ESF 11 does not have the requisite expertise to render appropriate assistance.

ESF 8 will assist ESF 11 as required to protect the health of livestock and companion and service animals by ensuring the safety of the manufacture and distribution of foods and drugs given to animals used for human food production. ESF

8 supports DHS/FEMA together with ESF 6 (Mass Care, Emergency Assistance, Housing, and Human Services), ESF 9 (Search and Rescue), and ESF 11 to ensure an integrated response to provide for the safety and well-being of household pets and service and companion animals.

ESF 8 supports ESF 6 by providing expertise and guidance on the public health issues of the medical needs populations.

4.7.5 National Disaster Medical System (NDMS, DMATs, DMORTs, MMRS)

The NDMS is a federally coordinated system that augments the nation's medical response capability. The overall purpose of the NDMS is to supplement an integrated national medical response capability for assisting state and local authorities in dealing with the medical impacts of major peacetime disasters and to provide support to the military and the VA medical systems in caring for casualties evacuated back to the United States from overseas armed conventional conflicts.[20]

The NRF utilizes the NDMS, as part of the HHS Office of Preparedness and Response, under ESF 8, Health and Medical Services, to support federal agencies in the management and coordination of the federal medical response to major emergencies and federally declared disasters, including:

➤ Natural disasters

➤ Major transportation accidents

➤ Technological disasters

➤ Acts of terrorism including weapons of mass destruction events

NDMS personnel are organized into five different teams: Disaster Medical Assistance Teams (DMATs), Disaster Mortuary Teams (DMORTs), National Veterinary Response Team (NVRT), National Nurse Response Team (NNRT), and National Pharmacy Response Teams (NPRTs). These assets are supplemented by the FEMA-operated Metropolitan Medical Response System (MMRS). The DMORT system was described in Section 4.6.10, and DMATs and the MMRS are described below.

Disaster Medical Assistance Team.   The DMAT is a group of professional and paraprofessional medical personnel (supported by a cadre of logistical and administrative staff) designed to provide medical care during a disaster or other event. NDMS recruits personnel for specific vacancies, plans for training opportunities, and coordinates the deployment of the team. To supplement the standard DMATs, there are highly specialized DMATs that deal with specific medical conditions such as crush injury, burns, pediatric emergencies, and mental health emergencies.[21]

DMATs are designed to be a rapid-response element to supplement local medical care until other federal or contract resources can be mobilized, or the situation is resolved. DMATs deploy to disaster sites with sufficient supplies and equipment to sustain themselves for a period of 72 hours while providing medical care at a fixed or temporary medical care site. Generally, the personnel are activated for a period of 2 weeks.

In mass casualty incidents, their responsibilities may include triaging patients, providing high-quality medical care despite the adverse and austere environment often found at a disaster site, patient reception at staging facilities, and preparing patients for evacuation.

Under the rare circumstance that disaster victims are evacuated to a different locale to receive definitive medical care, DMATs may be activated to support patient reception and disposition of patients to hospitals. DMATs are principally a community resource available to support local, regional, and state requirements. However, as a national resource they can be federalized.

Metropolitan Medical Response System.   On July 10, 1995, the USPHS Office of Emergency Preparedness and state and local EMS agencies released the first documents that pointed to the concept of a metropolitan medical strike team. This concept, through development and evolution, eventually became the MMRS.[22] The purpose was to review concepts and challenges of a medical response to an act of terrorism.

Consistent with the need to ensure effective and appropriate consequence management for nuclear, biologic, and chemical events, which are overwhelmingly medical in nature, the MMRS sought to resolve the present inability of civilian prehospital EMS agencies to minimize the effects of such attacks.

It was decided that MMRS jurisdictions must plan to mitigate the medical consequences of a weapons of mass destruction event by creating a highly trained, readily deployable, fully equipped response system of medical, law enforcement, fire service, and other professionals to support local resources.

Positioned at major 45 metropolitan areas, the MMRS serves the following essential functions:

➤ Chemical, biologic, or nuclear agent identification

➤ Medical intelligence gathering and distribution

➤ Patient triage and treatment capability and support

➤ Patient decontamination capability and support

➤ Coordination of patient transportation to receiving facilities

4.7.6   Laboratory Response Network (LRN)

The LRN is charged with the task of maintaining an integrated network of state and local public health, federal, military, and international laboratories that can respond to bioterrorism, chemical terrorism, and other public health emergencies.[23] The LRN is a unique asset in the nation's growing preparedness for biologic and chemical terrorism. The linking of state and local public health laboratories with veterinary, agriculture, military, and water- and food-testing laboratories is unprecedented.

4.7.7   Strategic National Stockpile (SNS)

The SNS, a program of the CDC, is a national repository of antibiotics, chemical antidotes, antitoxins, life-support medications, intravenous administration materials, airway maintenance supplies, and medical/surgical items. The SNS is designed to supplement and resupply state and local public health agencies in the event of a national emergency anywhere and at any time within the United States or its territories.[24]

The SNS is organized for flexible response. The first line of support lies within the immediate-response 12-hour "push packages." These are caches of pharmaceuticals, antidotes, and medical supplies designed to provide rapid delivery of a broad spectrum of assets for an ill-defined threat in the early hours of an event. These push packages are positioned in strategically located, secure warehouses ready for immediate deployment to a designated site within 12 hours of the federal decision to deploy SNS assets.

If the incident requires additional pharmaceuticals and/or medical supplies, follow-on vendor-managed inventory (VMI) supplies will be shipped to arrive within 24 to 36 hours. If the agent is well defined, VMI can be tailored to provide pharmaceuticals, supplies, and/or products specific to the suspected or confirmed agent(s). In this case, the VMI could act as the first option for immediate response from the SNS program.

4.7.8   USPHS Commissioned Corps

The USPHS Commissioned Corps is a team of more than 6000 full-time, well-trained, highly qualified public health professionals dedicated to delivering the nation's public health promotion and disease prevention programs and advancing public health science. As one of America's seven uniformed services, the Commissioned Corps fills essential public health leadership and service roles within the nation's federal government agencies and programs. The Corps has officers in many professions, including physicians, dentists, nurses, pharmacists, dietitians, engineers, environmental health officers, mental health specialists, health services officers, scientific researchers, a variety of therapists, and veterinarians. Commissioned Corps emergency response teams are managed by the Office of the Surgeon General. They are trained and equipped to respond to public health crises and national emergencies, such as natural disasters, disease outbreaks, or terrorist attacks. The teams are multidisciplinary and are capable of responding to domestic and international humanitarian missions.[25]

4.8 ROLE OF STATE AND REGIONAL DISASTER RESPONSE ENTITIES

State health departments work in conjunction with other state and local assets in responding to a disaster, especially when the event involves several local municipalities. In these situations, the state public health department may take the lead role in organizing the response.

When incidents are large or cross state lines, interstate compacts may come into play. Interstate compacts involve prearranged agreements to offer assistance to other states, including fire, police, and health care assets. It is imperative that these compacts, and the personnel who will implement them, be in place and well drilled *before* a disaster strikes.

4.9 LOCAL DISASTER RESPONSE

The first response to any disaster is always the local response. Local fire and police assets are usually the first agencies to respond to a disaster with immediate impact, eg, explosions, large fires, or earthquakes. Similarly, local public health agencies are typically the first health officials involved in disease outbreaks, including possible acts of bioterrorism.

However, many incidents may be beyond the scope of the local community's capacity to respond alone, the local community's capacity to respond alone, and local resources may be rapidly depleted. It is imperative, therefore, that local municipalities and states prepare for cooperation and joint response to a large incident. Again, these prearranged agreements must be practiced and drilled to ensure response operations. Waiting until a disaster occurs to find out who to call at the state level will invariably impede effective disaster response.

4.10 SUMMARY

Responsibility for an effective disaster response is shared by all members of the community, not a single agency or group. Resources needed to manage an event may become depleted. Cooperation among agencies and individuals is essential. This includes all levels of government and private sector responders. These agencies need to come together as a disaster health system and work efficiently and effectively together. This will eliminate duplication of effort, increase efficiency, and protect the safety of the entire community. Integral to an effective disaster health system is strong leadership and management, which can be achieved through the guidelines of the NIMS. Planning is also key to an effective response. All citizens should feel that they have a role to play in disaster response. In fact, personal preparedness and volunteerism may be key to a community's recovery.

4.11 SELF-LEARNING SCENARIOS

After completing the CDLS® course and each of the chapters in this manual, take time to work through the 4 scenarios presented in Appendix A. The scenarios are designed for the application and reinforcement of "core" concepts and principles in disaster life support.

REFERENCES

1. Regional ITS Architecture for Metropolitan Boston. http://www.eot.state.ma.us/regionalitsarchitecture/bostonv5/web/_stakeholders.htm. Accessed September 6, 2009.

2. Committee on Assuring the Health of the Public in the 21st Century, Institute of Medicine. *The Future of The Public's Health in the 21st Century*. Washington, DC: National Academies Press; 2003.

3. Public Health Functions Steering Committee. *Public Health in America*. July 1995. http://www.health.gov/phfunctions/public.htm. Accessed August 27, 2009.

4. Centers for Disease Control and Prevention. *Public Health's Infrastructure: A Status Report*. Washington, DC: US Department of Health and Human Services; 2001.

5. Department of Health and Human Services, Centers for Disease Control and Prevention. *Model Communities Link EMS and Public Health*. http://www.bt.cdc.gov/masscasualties/modelcommunities.asp. Accessed September 6, 2009.

6. Bell BP, Goldoft M, Griffin PM, et al. A multistate outbreak of *Escherichia coli* O157: H7-associated bloody diarrhea and hemolytic uremic syndrome from hamburgers: the Washington experience. *JAMA*. 1994;272:1349–1353.

7. Krohmer JR. *Principles of EMS Systems*. Dallas, TX: American College of Emergency Physicians; 2005.

8. National Registry of Emergency Medical Technicians. National EMS certification levels. http://www.nremt.org/Content/NREMT_Home.nremt. Accessed September 8, 2009.

9. Arch D, Zilm F, Berry R, Pietrzak M, Paeatore A. Integrating disaster preparedness and surge capacity in emergency facility planning. *J Ambulatory Care Manage*. 2008;31(4):377–385.

10. Cronin M, Lerner EB, Hise S, MacKenzie EJ, Teter H. *The Need for Linkages Between Public Health and the Trauma Care System In Disaster Response*. Upper Marlboro, MD: American Trauma Society; 2004.

11. Definitive care facilities. In: *Resources for the Optimal Care of the Injured Patient*. Chicago IL: American College of Surgeons; 2006.

12. Department of Homeland Security. *National Response Framework*. www.fema.gov/pdf/emergency/nrf/nrf-core.pdf. Accessed October 23, 2009.

13. Citizen Corps. Community Emergency Response Teams (CERT). http://www.citizencorps.gov/cert/. Accessed October 23, 2009.

14. Citizen Corps. Medical Reserve Corps. http://www.citizencorps.gov/programs/mrc_detailed.shtm. Accessed November 19, 2009.

15. Covello VT. Risk perception, risk communication, and EMF exposure: tools and techniques for communicating risk information. In: Matthes R, Bernhardt JH, Repacholi MH, eds. *Risk Perception, Risk Communication, and Its Application to EMF Exposure: Proceedings of the World Health Organization/ICNRP International Conference (ICNIRP 5/98)*. Vienna, Austria: International Commission on Non-Ionizing Radiation Protection; 1998:179–214.

16. Homeland Security Presidential Directive/HSPD-21. http://www.fas.org/irp/offdocs/nspd/hspd-21.htm. Accessed October 23, 2009.

17. Department of Homeland Security, FEMA. NIMS Resource Center. http://www.fema.gov/emergency/nims. Accessed September 5, 2009.

18. Department of Homeland Security, FEMA. Emergency Support Function #8 – Public Health and Medical Services Annex. http://www.fema.gov/pdf/emergency/nrf/nrf-esf-08.pdf. Accessed September 6, 2009.

19. US Public Health Service Commissioned Corps. Rapid Deployment Forces. http://ccrf.hhs.gov/ccrf/FactSheets/RDF_Fact_Sheet_Final.pdf. Accessed October 25, 2009.

20. Department of Health and Human Services, Assistant Secretary for Preparedness and Response. National Disaster Medical System (NDMS). http://www.hhs.gov/aspr/opeo/ndms/index.html. Accessed September 7, 2009.

21. Department of Health and Human Services, Assistant Secretary for Preparedness and Response. Disaster Medical Assistance Teams (DMAT). http://www.hhs.gov/aspr/opeo/ndms/teams/dmat.html. Accessed September 7, 2009.

22. Department of Homeland Security. FY 2009 Overview, Metropolitan Medical Response System. http://www.fema.gov/txt/government/grant/hsgp/fy09_hsgp_overview.txt. Accessed September 8, 2009.

23. Department of Health and Human Services, Centers for Disease Control and Prevention. The Laboratory Response Network Partners in Preparedness. http://www.bt.cdc.gov/lrn/. Accessed September 8, 2009.

24. Department of Health and Human Services, Centers for Disease Control and Prevention, Coordinating Office for Terrorism Preparedness and Emergency Response (COTPER). Strategic National Stockpile (SNS). http://emergency.cdc.gov/stockpile/index.asp. Accessed September 8, 2009.

25. Department of Health and Human Services. America's Health Responders: US Public Health Service Commissioned Corps. http://www.usphs.gov/. Accessed September 8, 2009.

CHAPTER FIVE

Public Health Law and Ethics

5.1 PURPOSE

This chapter identifies legal and ethical issues that impact disaster preparedness, including the basic legal framework for public health.*

5.2 LEARNING OBJECTIVES

After completing this chapter, readers will be able to:

➤ Given a disaster or public health emergency scenario, identify ethical issues that could be encountered by health professionals and other responders.

➤ Given a disaster or public health emergency scenario, identify legal and regulatory issues that may affect the ability of health professionals and others to render assistance.

➤ Given a disaster or public health emergency scenario, identify police powers that may be used by local authorities to protect public health and safety.

➤ Given a list of legislation and legal terms relevant to disasters and public health emergencies, match each with the most appropriate description.

---

*This chapter provides general information to assist emergency responders and health professionals in rendering assistance during a disaster. This includes having an understanding of the public health legal preparedness framework. The chapter does not constitute professional legal advice. Legal authorities and requirements vary by jurisdiction. Questions regarding legal matters should be directed to a licensed attorney.

5.3 DISASTER MEDICINE AND PUBLIC HEALTH PREPAREDNESS COMPETENCIES ADDRESSED

This chapter addresses the following competencies as delineated in Appendix E of this manual.

➤ Describe ethical issues relevant to the management of individuals (of all ages), populations, and communities affected by a disaster or public health emergency.

➤ Describe legal and regulatory issues relevant to disasters and public health emergencies, including the basic legal framework for public health.

5.4 OPENING VIGNETTE

You are a practicing nurse, at work on a Saturday night in the adult intensive care unit of a major urban medical center. An emergency alert has just flashed on the television screen in the visitor waiting room indicating that a category 4 hurricane with sustained winds of 131 to 155 mph and wind gusts reaching 140 mph has just dramatically changed course and is now headed directly toward your coastal city. It is predicted to make landfall by mid-Sunday morning. As you and your coworkers begin to assess the potential impact and implications of this situation, you begin to wonder:

What patients need to be protected and to what level of safety? If the hospital sustains serious damage, how will patients continue to receive treatment, and in what priority? Will they need to be evacuated and, if so, who should be evacuated first? How should potentially limited supplies of medications, medical equipment, food, and water be allocated, and in what priority? Who is going to make these decisions?

The Joint Commission requires hospitals to develop emergency management plans to help ensure effective responses to emergencies. The hospital's General Counsel and compliance committee have been working to address these questions. The emergency alert means that everyone is about to become busier.

5.5 OVERVIEW OF PUBLIC HEALTH LEGAL PREPAREDNESS

A sound legal framework is essential to assess and justify public health actions and interventions. Public health laws attempt to balance individual freedoms and welfare with the common welfare. Examples are the enforcement of quarantine (overruling individual freedom of movement), use of privately owned buildings for hospitals, and compulsory vaccination or implementation of emergency shifts in essential services. The goal of these interventions is to prevent the spread of a disease, which benefits the common welfare but may limit an individual's freedom during the crisis.

Public health legal preparedness is a subset of public health preparedness and can be defined as "attainment by a public health system of specified legal benchmarks or standards essential to the preparedness of the public health system."[1] There are four core elements to public health legal preparedness: laws, competencies, coordination, and information (Figure 5-1).

➤ *Laws or legal authorities* include statutes, ordinances, judicial rulings, policies, executive orders, administrative rules and regulations, memoranda of understanding, and mutual aid agreements.

➤ *Competencies* refers to the abilities and skills of both public and private sector agents of public health legal preparedness in accessing and understanding the relevant laws and applying them to given health issues.

➤ *Coordination* refers to law-based action across multiple jurisdictions and within the constitutional and political framework.

➤ *Information* refers to the availability of resources for use by agents in shaping and applying public health laws.

To enable emergency response efforts, the Centers for Disease Control and Prevention (CDC) supports promulgation of the Model State Emergency Health Powers Act, drafted by the Center for Law and the Public's Health at Georgetown and Johns Hopkins Universities.[2,3] The Act addresses four key areas: (1) emergency planning, (2) coordination among health care and public health systems, (3) control of property, and (4) personal care issues including vaccination, testing, therapy, isolation, and quarantine. These are effective powers that public health authorities may need to invoke in cases of potential mass casualties. Authorities are authorized to invoke these powers, taking into consideration individual liberties. The Act provides model language for the delineation of public health powers over property and protection of persons and the community in a consistent and uniform fashion.

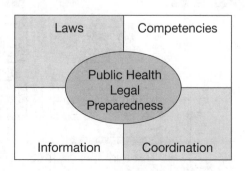

FIGURE 5-1

Resources on Legal Preparedness for Public Health Emergencies

Together with the CDC Public Health Law Program, the Association of State and Territorial Health Officials, and the National Association of County and City Health Officials, the Center for Law and the Public's Health at Georgetown and Johns Hopkins Universities prepared "Checklists on Legal Preparedness for Public Health Emergencies" that public health authorities can use to assess three important components of legal preparedness:

1. Interjurisdictional legal coordination for public health emergency preparedness

2. Local public health emergency legal preparedness and response

3. Civil legal liability related to public health emergencies

The checklists are available at http://www.publichealthlaw.net/Resources/BTlaw.htm.

Additional information on legal preparedness is available from the CDC Public Health Law Program at http://www2a.cdc.gov/phlp/index.asp.

5.6   SOURCES OF POWER AND LIMITS

The US Constitution provides a legal basis for public health law (Figure 5-2). Powers granted to the federal government include interstate commerce, national defense, and the power to tax and spend for public welfare. Powers reserved for the states include police power, which is defined as the authority of a government to impose restrictions on private rights and to enact measures to protect the health, safety, and welfare of their citizens. Included within the police powers is the authority of a state to act to protect the public's health. Public health powers within the Constitutional framework include surveillance, reporting, epidemiologic investigation, vaccination (voluntary or involuntary), isolation (voluntary or involuntary), treatment (voluntary or involuntary), social distancing measures, evacuation, and powers over property.

FIGURE 5-2

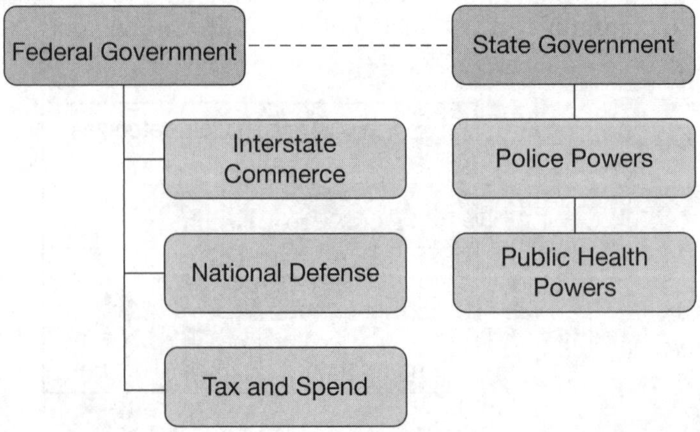

While almost all emergencies or disasters start locally, as the situation escalates local authorities may seek assistance from the state. Similarly, when a situation is beyond the capacity of a state, the state governor may request assistance from the US President through the Stafford Act.[4] When a disaster crosses state or national boarders, it falls within the purview of the federal government under the authority of the commerce clause. International agencies, particularly the World Health Organization (WHO), also play a role in protecting the population from infectious disease. While the WHO itself does not have quarantine authority, the International Health Regulations (IHR) provide the WHO with the responsibility of collecting international disease outbreak information and issuing advisories regarding travel when appropriate.[5]

The authority granted to government to protect the public's health is not without limits. Actions taken for the common good to protect the public's health must be balanced against individual liberties and needs. For example, in implementing quarantine and isolation measures, the basic needs (eg, food, medical care, safety, sanitation) of those who are confined must be met. Furthermore, some state laws may require confinement through the least restrictive means, such as in an individual's residence or other public or private premises.

5.7 DISEASE AND INJURY REPORTING

Every state has laws that require physicians to report certain diseases and injuries to a local or state health officer. Many extend this requirement to nurses, dentists, veterinarians, laboratories, school officials, institution administrators, and police officials. State laws require reporting of some or all communicable diseases, vital events such as births and deaths, cancer, and occupational and environmental conditions and injuries. Some state reporting systems are based on state laws and regulations adopted by the state board or department of health (which derives its authority from acts of the state legislature). Under certain emergency situations, surveillance activities may be initiated with additional reporting requirements that may be justified by the general charge to, and powers of, state and local public health agencies to protect the public health. Many of these reporting programs form the basis of modern public health preparedness sentinel warning systems.

Increasingly, efforts are being directed at collecting public health information in electronic formats such as from computerized clinical laboratory reports, medical record systems, and managed care databases. Despite these advances, the need for direct involvement of clinicians continues for immediate reporting of clinical syndromes, unusual disease presentations, and disease clusters in order to trigger a rapid public health response. Public health authorities are working toward a viable reporting system that will operate 24 hours a day, 7 days a week.

5.8 PRIVACY PROTECTION

An essential aspect of designing a disease and injury reporting system is to ensure that the privacy rights of persons whose information is of interest will not be violated. All states have statutes or regulations that provide some level of privacy protection for individual medical records and for health-related data maintained by the government. During a disaster event, the need to enhance public health surveillance capabilities and the need to communicate the resulting information can be confounded by the need to protect patient privacy. Disaster victims have reasonable rights to privacy regarding their bodies as well as information about themselves. Legal assurances of confidentiality are necessary to balance the public good that comes from surveillance with the privacy of individuals from whom data are collected.

The conflict between the "right to privacy" and the "need to know" concerning health care data must be monitored and addressed by any health surveillance program and is covered in existing federal legislation. For public health surveillance, the Health Insurance Portability and Accountability Act of 1996 (HIPAA) provides for the disclosure of patient data to appropriate authorities. The HIPAA Privacy Rule recognizes that various agencies and public officials will need protected health information to deal effectively with a disaster or other public health emergency.[6] To facilitate the communications that are essential to a quick and effective response to such events, the HIPAA Privacy Rule permits covered entities to disclose needed information to public officials in a variety of ways. Covered entities include health plans, health care clearinghouses (eg, billing services), and health professionals who transmit health information in electronic form in connection with certain transactions. In general, patient identifiers, except age and sex, should not be broadcast in any medium without clear patient consent. Assurances must be made that electronic systems to collect and store surveillance data and disseminate surveillance findings do not pose a risk to patient confidentiality.

The HIPAA Privacy Rule is not suspended in the event of a disaster or public health emergency.[7] However, the Health and Human Services (HHS) Secretary may waive sanctions and penalties against hospitals that do not comply with certain provisions, including (1) the patient's right to request privacy restrictions and (2) the patient's right to request confidential communications. Health professionals and health plans can share patient information for the purpose of providing treatment; locating or identifying individuals; notifying family members of the location of their loved ones; and preventing or lessening an imminent threat to the health and safety of a person or the public.[8] Entities not covered under the HIPAA Privacy Rule, such as the American Red Cross, are not restricted in sharing patient information.

5.9 DECLARATION OF A DISASTER OR PUBLIC HEALTH EMERGENCY

Declarations are both public announcements to inform the public of an event that may impact them and legal determinations made by an authorized government official. A declaration of a disaster or public health emergency triggers emergency powers, the expenditure of emergency funds, the activation of emergency plans, and suspension of certain regulatory statutes. Declarations may be made on the state and/or federal level and may be made for a general emergency, disaster, or public health emergency.

State law determines who can declare a disaster and what powers are conveyed to whom under that declaration. State statutes may provide for a declaration of a general emergency or disaster, which is often broadly defined as an occurrence that immediately threatens public health and/or safety. On the federal level, the HHS Secretary can declare a public health emergency under Section 319 of the Public Health Service Act.[9] A declaration may also be made by the US President under the Stafford Act. Declarations under the Stafford Act can be either at the request of a state or unilateral (without the request of a state) if the United States has exclusive or preeminent authority (eg, federal facilities, tribal lands).

5.10 EMERGENCY PUBLIC HEALTH POWERS

The power to implement measures necessary to protect the public's health is granted to each state under the US Constitution. These measures seek to balance individual rights and freedoms with the common welfare (eg, that of the general population). In a disaster or public health emergency, states have authority to exert reasonable control over citizens to directly secure and promote the welfare of the state and its people. The power to act in the best interests of the people provides states and municipalities with broad discretion in how they respond to a disaster situation. This includes possible encroachment on civil rights of people in the affected area to promote the public welfare.

Once a disaster or an emergency situation has been declared by the municipal authorities, there are several orders that may be issued on the basis of the police power available to the locality. These may include:

➤ Enforcing safety and sanitary codes

➤ Conducting inspections

➤ Requiring health professionals to report certain diseases to state authorities

➤ Establishing curfews

➤ Controlling entry into and out of the community

➤ Closing schools and businesses

➤ Ordering the evacuation of buildings, streets, neighborhoods, and cities

➤ Closing access to buildings, streets, or other public or private areas

➤ Imposing travel restrictions

➤ Controlling ingress and egress to and from a disaster area

➤ Controlling movement or persons within a disaster area

➤ Suspending the sale or dispensing of alcoholic beverages

➤ Suspending or limiting the sale, dispensing, or transportation of firearms, explosives, or combustibles

➤ Authorizing the acquisition or destruction of property, supplies, and materials

➤ Issuing orders for the disposal of corpses

The declaration of a public health emergency also may require special powers to protect public health and safety. These include the power to:

➤ Implement medical protocols and procedures to limit the spread of a disease (eg, mandatory vaccinations)

➤ Isolate and quarantine persons

➤ Access and disclose protected health information

➤ License and appoint health professionals

Isolation and Quarantine

Isolation and quarantine are two of the oldest public health interventions, dating back centuries. The purpose of both interventions is to decrease the number of individuals exposed to a contagious disease.

➤ *Isolation* is the placement of persons known to have a communicable disease in a separate area where they will not expose others.

➤ *Quarantine* is the placement of persons exposed to a contagious disease, but currently asymptomatic, in a separate area where they will not expose others and can be monitored for the development of the disease. Quarantine is required for several infectious diseases, such as smallpox and severe acute respiratory syndrome (SARS), because individuals can be contagious before the development of the signs and symptoms of the disease. During this asymptomatic but contagious period, they can potentially infect a large number of people.

While these measures may benefit the population in a public health emergency, state and local health authorities should review statutes, regulations, and ordinances that authorize these emergency measures and ensure legally sound procedures for executing them. It is important that public health authorities understand the legal and ethical implications of these emergency powers in order to implement them effectively and in a reasonable manner to limit infringement on individual rights and liberties.

5.11 LEGAL AND REGULATORY ISSUES IMPACTING HEALTH PROFESSIONALS IN A DISASTER

Disaster situations often involve mobilization of large numbers of health personnel from many states, raising questions about the "practice of medicine" and scope of practice in jurisdictions where an individual is not licensed. Verifying a provider's license and credentials has legal implications both for health care volunteers and for hospitals using their services. Health professionals should be aware of prohibitive challenges that exist in current government policies with regard to medical liability, standards of care, and license reciprocity to enable them to participate as volunteers in disaster response. While the commonly held "Good Samaritan Doctrine" is designed to encourage people to stop and render aid to those in need, each state recognizes the duties and potential liabilities under this doctrine somewhat differently.

5.11.1 License Reciprocity

Many states have adopted interstate mutual aid agreements, such as the Emergency Management Assistance Compact, which allow for volunteer health professionals licensed in one state to practice in another during a declared disaster. Similarly, the Uniform Emergency Volunteer Health Practitioners Act provides licensure reciprocity for volunteer health professionals who are registered with systems capable of confirming that persons are licensed and in good standing.[10] One such registry, the Emergency System for Advance Registration of Volunteer Health Professionals (ESAR-VHP), is a standardized state-based registration system sponsored by the HHS Office of the Assistant Secretary for Preparedness and Response.[11]

In addition to use of the ESAR-VHP, it is becoming a standard that responders are "cleared" and work through entities such as the Medical Reserve Corps, the National Disaster Medical System, and/or state medical response teams. Such entities perform the background screening and provide a framework of core knowledge that is required before a volunteer may function as an official member of a team sent to respond to a disaster.

5.11.2   Scope of Practice and "Standards of Care"

While many states provide for licensure reciprocity, volunteer health care professionals are usually not authorized to provide services outside of their scope of practice, even if similarly licensed practitioners in the states would be permitted to provide the services. The standard of care owed to a patient by a health professional depends on the circumstances. What is deemed to be "reasonable" care under normal circumstances may not be feasible during a serious disaster or public health emergency, in which large numbers of injured or ill persons overwhelm existing health system capacities and capabilities. Federal agencies and health organizations are developing guidance and policy related to adjusting the standard of care in a mass casualty event.[12-14]

5.11.3   Liability Concerns for Volunteer Health Care Professionals

The risk of civil and criminal liability during emergencies is one of the primary concerns of health professionals in responding to a disaster. During a disaster, health professionals may be liable for negligent or intentional acts that cause harm to a patient. Immunity from civil liability may be available through (1) governmental sovereign immunity (if the worker or volunteer is a government employee or agent), (2) federal and state volunteer protection acts, (3) Good Samaritan statutes, (4) state emergency health powers statutes, and (5) mutual aid compacts. However, the protections and regulations available to health professionals vary greatly by state and often depend on the health professional's method of deployment or status as a volunteer or employee. There is no immunity available for acts that may give rise to criminal liability.

5.11.4   Workers' Compensation

All states and the federal government have enacted workers' compensation laws to provide limited benefits to victims of work-related injuries or death, regardless of fault. The application of workers' compensation benefits to those who are injured while responding to a disaster depends on the responders' status as employees or volunteers, their employers, and the state or federal law that applies to them. Most workers' compensation laws cover only employees, but some states may legislatively extend coverage to include volunteer workers. In many jurisdictions, a volunteer's existing employer will not be liable for the injuries an employee sustains in providing services outside the course of employment. Several state laws define volunteers as employees of the state during a disaster. In these states, volunteers may be eligible for benefits from the institution for which they are temporarily employed.

5.12 MORAL AND ETHICAL CONSIDERATIONS IN DISASTERS

The application of ethical theories is necessary to establish a code of moral conduct and provide a framework to guide those involved in disaster planning, response, and recovery. Decisions made in a disaster situation will impact the health and lives of individuals and populations and are thus fundamentally moral in nature. Policies, such as those that guide the allocation of scarce resources or limit an individual's liberty, may adversely impact segments of the population, thereby reducing the public's confidence and trust in decision makers. A lack of public trust may ultimately hinder compliance or cooperation with advice or orders, which is necessary for an effective response to a disaster situation. Ensuring that these difficult decisions are based on sound scientific and ethical principles and that health professionals and other responders act in accord with these standards will help to build and maintain public confidence and trust in a disaster.

In a disaster, ethics is closely intertwined with the legal framework that will be used to guide policy decisions. During the disaster planning process, it will become clear that serious moral and ethical issues must be confronted before, during, and after an event. To help address these issues, ethics provides four broad basic principles to guide policy development and decision making in a disaster[15]:

➤ The *principle of autonomy* focuses on people's right to self-determination, the need to justify infringements on individual rights, and the need to balance individuals' freedoms should they compete and/or conflict.

➤ The *principle of beneficence* establishes a duty to promote individual and public welfare through the maximizing of benefits and minimizing of harms.

➤ The *principle of nonmaleficence* directs health professionals to actively avoid harming patients and communities.

➤ The *principle of justice* requires equitable distribution of benefits and risks.

In the process of ethical analysis and decision making, these four principles must work in concert. While all ethical principles are considered to be of equal importance, certain situations may invoke the use of certain principles to a greater or lesser extent. In some situations, a specific principle rightly takes primacy over other considerations. When treating patients, for example, the principle of beneficence is most directly relevant and serves as a health professional's chief consideration.

At the community level, these ethical principles can be invoked to balance individual and population needs to maximize public health benefits while respecting individual rights (to the greatest extent possible). The application of ethical principles to public health policy necessitates that responders provide for the health needs of all affected persons without regard to age, race, ethnicity, nationality, religious beliefs, sexual orientation, residency status, or socioeconomic status. While age may be a consideration when medical needs and probable outcomes are assessed, it cannot be the sole or dominating decision-making criterion.

Ethical Considerations to Guide Decisions in Disasters and Public Health Emergencies

The application of ethical principles to disaster preparedness and response leads to the development of a specific set of considerations to guide those who directly and indirectly participate in decision making:

Respect Persons and Communities

Ensure that disaster-related policies are consistent with the values of the community and protect all persons within the community. Members of the public must be allowed to participate and provide input into the disaster planning process. Circumstances such as poor community meeting attendance or poor community response to published policies may cause the interests of minorities (such as the elderly or individuals at a lower socioeconomic level) to be inadequately represented. The "stronger" populations tend to be more vocal and have the time to express and promote their values. Thus, "community" values may not accurately reflect actual consensus values.

Protect the Public From Harm

When serious, clear, and imminent harm is foreseeable, public health authorities should act to protect the health and well-being of the public. Appropriate interventions must be selected on the basis of their anticipated benefits to the public and weighed against foreseeable risks.

Provide Care

Health professionals have an ethical responsibility to take care of those in need in emergency situations, even when doing so may pose some risk to their own health. In a disaster, health professionals also must preserve their ability to meet victims' needs and are therefore advised against exposing themselves to unnecessary dangers.

Maintain Transparency

The development of disaster-related policies should be undertaken in a way that is transparent to the public. Members of the community should understand how policies are developed and how the policies impact the community, and they should be given the opportunity to comment during the policymaking process. Policies should be based on the best available scientific evidence.

Communicate Openly

The public is entitled to honest, accurate information about public health issues that affect them. This information should include the risks and benefits of their options.

Promote Equity

When resources are inadequate to meet the needs of the population, access must be appropriate and based on rational criteria. Decisions regarding the distribution of benefits and burdens must be made by fairly weighing risks, benefits, and costs. These decisions may in turn need to be reassessed and reevaluated as situations change and new information becomes available.

In times of resource scarcity, it is not uncommon for individuals to sacrifice a resource for the sake of others if they are made aware of the situation and presented with the opportunity.

Act With Proportionality

When the use of governmental power can be justified to protect public health, that power should be exercised in a way that avoids unnecessary impact on individuals and community groups.

Respect Individual Liberty

During nonemergencies, individuals have the right to travel, assemble freely, refuse treatment, and be secure in their person without restraint or compulsion. In a disaster or public health emergency, these liberties may be limited temporarily in the face of an overwhelming public interest. Any infringement on personal liberties must be minimized and subject to appropriate due process protections.

Protect Privacy

Individuals have the right to privacy of information about their health condition unless the disclosure of confidential information serves a clear, important public health objective and follows applicable law. When public health reporting is necessary, only the minimum information should be disclosed to minimize infringement on individual privacy rights.

Act With Reciprocity

When health professionals, patients, and their families face a disproportionate burden to protect public health, there is a societal obligation to take reasonable steps to minimize the burden.

Protect Against Stigmatization

Public health officials should act to minimize harm to groups and individuals who may be at risk due to hostile or discriminatory behavior during a disaster or public health emergency.

Source: Adapted from CDC[16] and New Mexico Department of Health.[17]

5.13 SUMMARY

In a crisis, state and local public health leaders need a clearly defined set of legal and ethical principles to help them make sound, real-time decisions for managing the situation and allocating potentially scarce resources. The all-hazards approach to public health preparedness requires that these principles be adaptable to a variety of emergencies, ranging from disease pandemics to terrorism to weather-related events.

5.14   SELF-LEARNING SCENARIOS

After completing the CDLS course and each of the chapters in this manual, take time to work through the 4 scenarios presented in Appendix A. The scenarios are designed for the application and reinforcement of "core" concepts and principles in disaster life support.

REFERENCES

1. Moulton AD, Gottfried RN, Goodman RA, Murphy AM, Rawson RD. What is public health legal preparedness? *J Law Med Ethics*. 2003;31:672–683.

2. Gostin LO, Sapsin JW, Teret S, et al. The Model State Emergency Health Powers Act: planning and response to bioterrorism and naturally occurring infectious disease. *JAMA*. 2002;288:622–628. http://jama.ama-assn.org/cgi/content/full/288/5/622. Accessed July 10, 2009.

3. Model State Emergency Health Powers Act. http://www.publichealthlaw.net/MSEHPA/MSEHPA.pdf. Accessed July 10, 2009.

4. Robert T. Stafford Disaster Relief and Emergency Assistance Act (Public Law 93-288) as amended. http://www.fema.gov/about/stafact.shtm. Accessed July 10, 2009.

5. World Health Organization. *International Health Regulations*. Geneva, Switzerland: World Health Organization; 2005. http://www.who.int/csr/ihr/en/. Accessed July 10, 2009.

6. HIPAA Privacy Rule and public health: guidance from the Centers for Disease Control and Prevention and the U.S. Department of Health and Human Services. *MMWR*. 2003;52:1–12. http://www.cdc.gov/mmwr/preview/mmwrhtml/m2e411a1.htm. Accessed July 10, 2009.

7. Department of Health and Human Services. HIPAA Frequent Questions: Is the HIPAA Privacy Rule suspended during a national or public health emergency? http://www.hhs.gov/hipaafaq/providers/hipaa-1068.html. Accessed July 10, 2009.

8. Department of Health and Human Services, Office for Civil Rights. Hurricane Katrina Bulletin: HIPAA Privacy and Disclosures in Emergency Situations. September 2, 2005. Available at http://www.hhs.gov/ocr/privacy/hipaa/understanding/special/emergency/katrinahipaa.pdf. Accessed November 19, 2009.

9. Public Health Service Act. http://www.fda.gov/RegulatoryInformation/Legislation/ucm148717.htm. Accessed July 10, 2009.

10. Uniform Emergency Volunteer Health Practitioners Act. http://www.uevhpa.org/DesktopDefault.aspx?tabindex=1&tabid=55. Accessed July 10, 2009.

11. Health Resources and Services Administration. *Emergency System for Advance Registration of Volunteer Health Professionals (ESAR-VHP): Legal and Regulatory Issues*. Draft report. Washington, DC: US Department of Health and Human Services; 2006. http://www.publichealthlaw.net/Research/PDF/ESAR%20VHP%20Report.pdf. Accessed July 10, 2009.

12. Agency for Healthcare Research and Quality. *Altered Standards of Care in Mass Casualty Events: Bioterrorism and Other Public Health Emergencies*. Publication 05-0043. Rockville, MD: AHRQ; 2005. http://www.ahrq.gov/research/altstand/. Accessed July 9, 2009.

13. Center for Health Policy, Columbia University School of Nursing. *Adapting Standards of Care Under Extreme Conditions: Guidance for Professionals During Disasters,*

Pandemics, and Other Extreme Emergencies. Washington, DC: American Nurses Association; 2008.

14. Guidance for Establishing Crisis Standards of Care for Use in Disaster Situations: A Letter Report. Bruce M. Altervogt, Clare Stroud, Sarah L. Hanson, Dan Hanfling, and Lawrence O. Gostin, Editors. Committee on Guidance for Establishing Standards of Care for Use in Disaster Situations; Institute of Medicine. http:www.nap.edu/catalog/12749.html. Accessed October 22, 2009.

15. Beauchamp T, Childress J. *Principles of Biomedical Ethics.* 5th ed. New York, NY: Oxford University Press; 2001.

16. Ethics Subcommittee of the Advisory Committee to the Director, Centers for Disease Control and Prevention. *Ethical Guidelines in Pandemic Influenza.* Atlanta: Centers for Disease Control and Prevention; 2007. http://www.cdc.gov/od/science/phethics/guidelinesPanFlu.htm. Accessed July 10, 2009.

17. New Mexico Department of Health, Bureau of Health Emergency Management. Original Pandemic Influenza Briefing and Resource Book, Part 5, Attachment 12: Ethics Guidance and Matrix; 2006. http://www.health.state.nm.us/ohem/opibr/Update%20Book%2052606%20part%205/Ethics%20Guidance%20and%20Matrix.pdf. Accessed November 17, 2008.

CHAPTER SIX

The DISASTER Paradigm™

6.1 PURPOSE

This chapter discusses the elements of the DISASTER Paradigm™ and the utility of this all-hazards framework for the management of disasters and other mass casualty events.

6.2 LEARNING OBJECTIVES

After completing this chapter, readers should be able to:

➤ Given a disaster or public health emergency scenario, identify early warning systems, indicators, and clues that may signal the onset of the event.

➤ Given a list of terms from the incident management lexicon, match each to its definition or description.

➤ Describe important health, safety, and security risks that should be considered at any disaster scene.

➤ Given a scenario involving exposure to a possible communicable disease, describe personal, institutional, and community protective measures to prevent and control the spread of the disease.

➤ Discuss the purpose and rationale for personal protective equipment at a disaster scene or receiving facility.

➤ Discuss the purpose and rationale for victim decontamination at a disaster scene or receiving facility.

➤ Define *surge capacity* in the context of health system response to disasters and public health emergencies.

➤ Given a mass casualty scenario, discuss the purpose of triage at the disaster scene and at receiving facilities.

➤ Identify basic lifesaving and life support measures that may be applied to minimize morbidity and mortality at the disaster scene.

➤ Given a disaster scenario, describe situations and circumstances that may hinder the safe evacuation of affected populations.

➤ Identify potential strategies to ensure the continuity of supplies and services to meet the immediate medical and mental health needs of displaced and nondisplaced persons and their families.

➤ Given a disaster or public health emergency scenario, describe the potential short- and long-term impact of the event on the recovery of the local health system.

6.3   DISASTER MEDICINE AND PUBLIC HEALTH PREPAREDNESS COMPETENCIES ADDRESSED

This chapter addresses the following competencies as delineated in Appendix E of this manual:

➤ Recognize general indicators and epidemiologic clues of a disaster or public health emergency (including natural, unintentional, and terrorist events).

➤ Describe the purpose and relevance of the National Response Framework (NRF), National Incident Management System (NIMS), Hospital Incident Command System (HICS), and emergency support function 8 to regional, community, and institutional disaster response.

➤ Describe the potential effect of mass casualties on access to and availability of clinical and public health resources in a disaster.

➤ Using an all-hazards framework, explain general health, safety, and security risks associated with disasters.

➤ Describe infection control precautions to protect health care workers, other responders, and the public from exposure to communicable diseases, such as pandemic influenza.

➤ Describe the rationale, function, and limitations of personal protective equipment that may be used in a disaster or public health emergency.

➤ Explain the purpose of victim decontamination in a disaster.

➤ Explain the role of triage as a basis for prioritizing or rationing health care services for victims and communities affected by a disaster or public health emergency.

➤ Explain basic lifesaving and support principles and procedures that can be used at a disaster scene.

➤ Describe solutions for ensuring the continuity of supplies and services to meet the medical and mental health needs of oneself, family, office practice, institution, and company in a disaster under various contingency situations (eg, mass evacuation, mass sheltering, prolonged shelter-in-place).

➤ Describe short- and long-term medical and mental health considerations for the recovery of all ages, populations, and communities affected by a disaster or public health emergency.

6.4 INTRODUCTION

The National Disaster Life Support™ (NDLS) Program is grounded on the application and promotion of a practical, all-hazards mnemonic called the DISASTER Paradigm.™ The all-hazards approach to disaster planning, training, and response emphasizes that the basic tenets of disaster management are the same, regardless of the cause of the disaster. Each letter in this paradigm applies to a key element in the health response to any mass casualty event. These elements are:

D Detection

I Incident management

S Safety and security

A Assess hazards

S Support

T Triage and treatment

E Evacuation

R Recovery

Overall, the DISASTER Paradigm provides:

➤ A uniform framework for addressing disaster recognition, response, and recovery

➤ An organizational tool for responders to assess individual and community needs and utilize available resources

➤ A mechanism for promoting the consistency of communications among emergency responders and response agencies

The Core Disaster Life Support® course provides an overview of the DISASTER Paradigm in the context of the all-hazards approach to disaster management. Application of this paradigm to specific emergency events, with more detailed discussion of clinical and public health implications, is addressed in the Basic Disaster Life Support™ (BDLS®) and Advanced Disaster Life Support™ (ADLS®) courses.

6.5   DETECTION

Detection is the initial recognition that a threat is imminent or exists. The key to detection of a disaster is ongoing vigilance and situational awareness of abnormal changes in the immediate environment, as well as awareness of unusual disease patterns and occurrences in the vicinity. Detection is not just about major emergencies—it may be simply identifying something outside the norm.

The goals of detection are to:

➤ Determine that a real emergency exists that may overwhelm immediately available resources

➤ Protect personal safety and prevent harm to others

➤ Determine the possible cause of the situation

➤ Declare the existence of the emergency or disaster to others so that they may respond appropriately

➤ Alert local authorities so that they can begin to plan for or initiate a rapid and coordinated response to save lives, protect property, and meet basic needs

6.5.1   Immediate Priorities

The top priority during the response to any disaster must always be personal protection. Specifically, one should reflect on the following questions:

➤ Does anything appear out of the ordinary?

➤ What possible hazards are present?

➤ What resources are available to help?

➤ What information can witnesses provide?

The detection process involves recognizing that a situation exists that could overwhelm the resources available. When it is evident that immediate response needs outweigh the available resources, a disaster exists. Actions taken in the following minutes and hours will become extremely important to protect the health, safety, and security of all affected populations. In such situations, it will be critical to communicate effectively with the emergency management and response organizations, hospitals, and the public health system.

6.5.2 Emergency Warning and Alert Systems

In the United States, federal agencies such as the National Oceanic and Atmospheric Administration (NOAA) and the US Geological Survey (USGS) constantly monitor for natural disaster threats. Despite their best efforts, the circumstances, severity, and exact strike point of some disasters are hard to reliably predict. Hurricanes can be identified and tracked for days before landfall, while lightning strikes and earthquakes occur with little or no warning.

Warning the public in the event of an emergency is a key function of local emergency management agencies. The timely notification of an impending threat or danger may help people take lifesaving actions and prevent widespread injuries. Advance warning and predictive forecasting systems have been developed by academic institutions and government agencies to detect some natural disasters (eg, hurricanes, earthquakes, tsunamis, and volcanic eruptions). Such systems facilitate disaster mitigation by allowing for more rapid implementation of emergency response plans and operations.

In the United States, the capacity to issue disaster warnings is provided primarily through the Emergency Alert System (EAS) and the NOAA Weather Radio All-Hazards Network, both of which rely primarily on broadcasting media.[1,2] The EAS is the successor to the Emergency Broadcast System (EBS), which began in 1964. It was upgraded in 1997 to include digital communications and automation technology and to eliminate several problems that developed with the EBS. The Federal Communications Commission mandates that the EAS be used only for warning of an imminent threat to life or property. If the EAS is activated, national, state, and local television and radio broadcast stations will deliver important emergency information to the public. The Federal Emergency Management Agency (FEMA) is responsible for national-level activation of the EAS as well as testing of the system.

The National Warning System (NAWAS) is a hardened communication system that was originally designed to allow the federal government to communicate with state civil defense and emergency management agencies to warn of an incoming nuclear attack. The NAWAS has become the backbone of a system that allows reliable communication from the federal government to state and local governments during major disasters.

The NOAA Weather Radio Network is a network of radio stations broadcasting continuous weather information directly from a nearby National

Weather Service (NWS) office. NOAA Weather Radio broadcasts severe weather warnings, watches, forecasts, and other hazard information 24 hours a day. More recently, the NOAA Weather Radio has been adapted to become an all-hazards emergency communication tool. Although used most often for weather threats, emergency management agencies can request the NWS to automatically sound an alarm on individual radio receivers and trigger cable television and broadcast media to display emergency messages. Whether communicating the presence of a chemical release, an impending tsunami, or an approaching tornado, this system provides valuable advance warning to those in harm's way and can reduce the number of victims from an event.

Given the advanced state of communication technologies, especially the Internet and wireless devices, the capability to deliver emergency warnings is being expanded beyond radio and television broadcasts. A number of states and communities are implementing alert systems that use e-mail, wireless text messages, or the Internet for alerts; some issue mass alerts to telephones by using autodialing technologies, or to wireless devices by using cellular broadcasting technology. In addition to emergency alert broadcasts, many communities utilize outdoor warning systems. Typically, these consist of a network of sirens and highway message boards that are activated by local authorities in an emergency.

6.5.3   Detection of Biologic Emergencies

Detection of a biologic emergency may be difficult, particularly if sick persons are distributed over wide geographic regions. It may take days or weeks before an exposure leads to observable signs and symptoms. Timely and accurate detection and confirmation of a disease outbreak requires a coordinated process, involving a team of health professionals. Typically, this is initiated by an alert clinician who recognizes an unusual clinical presentation in a patient, promptly reports the situation to public health authorities, and submits appropriate specimens for laboratory testing and analysis.

Biologic agents can enter the body through ingestion, inhalation, injection, and penetration through broken skin and mucous membranes (eyes, nose, or mouth). Signs and symptoms vary depending on the specific agent involved, the route of exposure, and the susceptibility of the victim to infection. The precise identification of some biologic agents may require specialized testing that takes several days.

Biologic agents may cause a variety of nonspecific influenza-like signs and symptoms, especially in the early phase of the illness (eg, fever, weakness and fatigue, cough, muscle aches, headache, sore throat). Timely and accurate diagnosis depends in large measure on the clinical presentation and exposure history, as well as on familiarity with the unique aspects of the disease. Symptoms may go unnoticed or may be attributed to less serious conditions unless or until atypical illness patterns and diagnostic clues become apparent.

Clues Suggestive of a Biologic Event [3, 4]

Suspicion should be raised when there appear to be many previously "healthy" people becoming sick or displaying an unusual pattern of symptoms. This includes the following situations:

ILLNESS OUT OF RANGE

➤ Sudden, unexplained increase in influenza (flu)-like illness in a short period of time, especially in young, otherwise healthy populations

➤ Sudden, unexplained cluster of patients with rash, pneumonia, bleeding, or death, or requiring hospital (especially intensive care unit) admission

➤ Sudden increase in seriousness or mortality associated with a seemingly common illness

➤ Sudden increase in the number of patient telephone calls for influenza, rash, neurologic symptoms, lower respiratory symptoms, or requests for antibiotics

ILLNESS OUT OF CONTEXT

➤ Outbreak of influenza-like illness in a well-immunized population

➤ Influenza-like illness associated with unusual complications, such as bleeding, pneumonia, acute respiratory distress syndrome, swollen lymph nodes, or rash

➤ Cluster of treatment failures in an illness that usually responds to therapy

ILLNESS OUT OF SEQUENCE

➤ Outbreak of illness affecting only one age group, gender, or ethnic group, or persons who work in a particular facility

➤ Clusters of human illness simultaneous with or immediately following reports of an outbreak of animal disease or death in the same geographic region

ILLNESS OUT OF SEASON

➤ Influenza outbreak in the late spring or summer

➤ Winter outbreak of an illness that is typically arthropod-borne (plague, typhus, Rocky Mountain spotted fever, tick- or mosquito-borne encephalitis)

ILLNESS OUT OF PLACE

➤ The occurrence of even one case of a potential disease in a location where it would not be expected to occur naturally. An exception would be in a person who has returned from an area endemic for that illness and the symptom onset began within the expected incubation period. Examples include even one case of Ebola hemorrhagic fever or smallpox in the United States.

One of the critical factors in a biologic emergency is the delay from exposure to symptom onset. Symptom onset may be delayed for days or weeks. As such, there may be no traditional "scene," where large numbers of exposed persons are concentrated in time and space. Rather an incubation period permits infected

---

BioSense

BioSense is a national program, coordinated by the Centers for Disease Control and Prevention (CDC), to improve national capabilities for conducting public health surveillance and to enable health situational awareness through access to existing data from health organizations across the country. Traditional public health surveillance and investigations often involve manual reporting of cases to public health agencies and telephone calls to health care providers for more detailed patient chart information. Such processes can be problematic, especially during a public health emergency.

Data analysis methods supported by BioSense address the need for real-time national surveillance and event detection and management, which are critical in containing and minimizing threats from infectious diseases, for biologic and chemical attacks, and for naturally occurring emergencies. BioSense was developed to support early event detection and represents an approach to public health surveillance based on electronic data received from numerous sources such as emergency departments, physician offices and clinics, pharmacies, and clinical laboratories.

More information on the BioSense Program is available at http://www.cdc.gov/BioSense/.

---

persons to move about, interact with others, and travel over wide geographic areas, increasing the risk of disease transmission.

Some biologic agents have a high potential for secondary transmission from infected persons to others. In a suspected outbreak, public health authorities should be notified as soon as possible so they can begin to plan and implement measures to control disease spread. Hospital, commercial, and public health laboratories are staffed by scientists, medical technologists, and technicians who analyze patient and environmental specimens for clues to the cause of the disease. Public health authorities have a responsibility to ensure access to laboratory services for the diagnostic testing required to support emergency health and medical services in a time-sensitive manner.

6.5.4   Detection of Chemical Emergencies

Once released, chemical agents can contaminate air, food, water, and consumer products, entering the body by ingestion, inhalation, injection, or absorption through the skin. Some chemical agents have a high potential for secondary contamination from exposed persons to responders, which requires that on-scene and other health personnel who treat these casualties take appropriate safety

Clues Suggestive of a Chemical Emergency[5]

Possible clues of a chemical release include:

➤ An unusual increase in the number of persons seeking care for a rapid onset of symptoms

➤ Rapid onset of illness with little or no warning

➤ Unexplained illness or death among young or previously healthy persons

➤ Presence of an unexplained odor, low-level clouds, or vapors at the scene

➤ Emission of unexplained odors from ill persons

➤ Clusters of illness in persons who have common characteristics, such as drinking water or eating food from the same source

➤ Unexplained death of plants, fish, or animals (domestic or wild)

➤ A syndrome (ie, a constellation of clinical signs and symptoms in patients) suggesting a disease commonly associated with a known chemical exposure

➤ Sudden unexplained weakness, collapse, apnea, or convulsions in previously healthy persons

➤ Dimmed or blurred vision

➤ Hypersecretion syndromes (eg, tearing, drooling, diarrhea)

➤ Inhalation syndromes (eye, nose, throat, chest irritation; shortness of breath)

➤ Burn-like syndromes (redness, blistering, itching, sloughing)

precautions. Most chemical exposures cause immediate symptoms, as opposed to biologic exposures, which have an incubation period. Therefore, when multiple victims present from the same location with the same time of onset of symptoms, a chemical exposure should be suspected.

Emergency workers and health personnel must consider the possibility of chemical agent exposure resulting from any mass casualty event. Safety may hinge on awareness of specific clues at the scene and knowledge of the symptoms that various chemicals may cause.

Various sensors and detectors are available commercially to monitor and identify chemical agents at or near release sites. A simple rapid detection method involves chemical detection paper that reacts with specific chemicals to produce a color change, similar to pH paper. Unfortunately, chemical papers are effective only when in direct contact with liquids or heavy vapors. Other detection systems rely on air sampling, such as Dräger tubes, the Advanced Portable Detector 2000, and other monitors, which can detect very low levels of chemicals. Proper use of these devices requires training and maintenance. As such, they are difficult for most hospitals and public health departments to maintain and operate but are widely used by fire departments and hazardous materials (HAZMAT) teams.

With a chemical release, responder safety and casualty survival hinge not only on awareness of clues at the scene, but also on knowledge and recognition of characteristic signs and symptoms of various chemicals and chemical classes. While some chemical agents may have a characteristic odor (eg, chlorine), real-time identification of most chemicals at a disaster scene may be impossible because the specialized detection equipment required may not be available. In addition, identification by smell requires exposure to the agent, and some hazardous materials (eg, phosgene, cyanide) cannot be reliably detected via smell.

Chemical agents most often produce signs and symptoms soon after exposure, typically within minutes or hours of the event. After exposure, nonspecific presentations may appear, including altered mental status (confusion), loss of consciousness, seizures, respiratory distress (trouble breathing), and cardiovascular collapse. Early symptoms of chemical exposure can include nausea, vomiting, and diarrhea (which also are symptoms of psychological stress). Clinical effects will vary depending on the:

➤ Type of agent

➤ Route of exposure

➤ Amount and concentration of agent

➤ Duration of exposure

➤ Preexisting medical conditions in the exposed individual

Each chemical class causes a typical, specific set of signs and symptoms called a *toxidrome* (a combination of the words "toxic," or poison, and "syndrome"). Knowledge of the major clinical syndromes or toxidromes caused by major classes of chemical agents may facilitate detection and treatment. If chemical detection devices are not available, emergency responders and health workers will need to begin treatment, and decontamination, for possible chemical exposure on the basis of clinical presentation. Chemical classes of concern to disaster responders include, but are not limited to:

➤ Pulmonary, irritant gases (choking agents) (eg, chlorine, phosgene, many industrial chemicals)

➤ Blister or vesicant agents (eg, sulfur mustard)

➤ Asphyxiant agents (eg, cyanide, carbon monoxide, hydrogen sulfide)

➤ Nerve agents (eg, sarin, VX)

➤ Incapacitating agents (eg, tear gas, pepper spray, 3-quinuclidinyl benzilate [BZ])

6.5.5   Detection of Radiation Emergencies

Without specialized equipment, the release of radioactive materials can be difficult to detect because most forms of radiation are odorless, colorless, and invisible. In the absence of an overt event (such as detonation of a "dirty" bomb or industrial plant catastrophe), detection of radiation exposure can be delayed and remote from the release site. Except in cases where persons are exposed to massive radiation doses, symptom onset may be delayed by hours to weeks or even longer. Detection of a radiologic event may rely on an astute clinician with an increased level of suspicion when examining a patient or reviewing a complete blood count with differential.

Detection of a major nuclear event will be obvious, because this type of detonation leads to the release of massive amounts of energy, with a resulting "mushroom cloud." The released energy will produce mostly blast energy, as well as heat, radiation, and fallout. If a person survives the physical trauma of the nuclear blast, the detection of acute radiation exposure will be the same as described for other radiation events.

A radiologic survey conducted with specialized equipment is the only way to confirm the presence of radiation. People exposed to a source of radiation can become ill if their dose is high enough, but they do not become radioactive. Radioactivity can be easily detected by a number of devices, such as Geiger-Mueller counters, dosimeters (sensors that measure the cumulative dose of radiation emitted by a radioactive source), radiation pagers, and other equipment. Geiger counters measure radiation coming from a source at a specific point in time. These instruments are important in detecting contamination and monitoring casualties for completeness of removal of radioactive material after decontamination procedures. The use of Geiger counters requires some training and proper calibration. Fortunately, most hospitals have these devices and trained personnel (health physicists) because of the use of nuclear medicine therapies that require radioactive material. Personal dosimeters, as the term suggests, measure the cumulative radiation dose to which a person has been exposed. These are rather inexpensive and more readily available.

Exposure to low levels of radiation is not likely to cause significant illness or injury, especially soon after an event. Exposed persons may have no symptoms, or, in the case of a dirty bomb, may display only traumatic injuries resulting from the primary explosion. The earlier the symptoms develop after exposure, the higher the dose to which the person was exposed (assuming the symptoms are caused by the radiation itself, not by other factors).

The initial symptoms after acute whole-body radiation doses are likely to include "prodromal symptoms" of nausea, vomiting, diarrhea, and potential behavioral changes. Vomiting within 2 hours of the event indicates a potentially significant radiation exposure. If diarrhea persists beyond 2 to 3 days, the outlook may be poor. (It must be noted that these symptoms can also be the result of psychological stress.)

If a person is believed to have received a high radiation dose, an immediate blood cell count, followed by additional blood examinations at 5 or 10 days, will give a clear indication of likelihood of survival or evidence that more serious attention to and treatment of the exposed person is needed. High levels of radiation exposure cause a wide range of signs and symptoms (called *acute radiation syndromes*) affecting all organ systems. Observable health effects generally occur soon after receipt of large doses; they include:

➤ Hair loss

➤ Skin burns

➤ Nausea

➤ Possible death

Skin effects of radiation exposure include itching and redness and can begin within hours of exposure to either large doses of total-body radiation or direct contact with a radioactive source (at lower doses, these symptoms may be delayed). Symptoms will subside for several days or weeks, and then intense reddening, itching, blistering, and ulceration will occur. These effects can be worsened by simultaneous thermal burns or traumatic injuries.

6.6 INCIDENT MANAGEMENT

Once an emergency situation has been detected, the safe and successful management of the event depends on the consistent application of core principals and proven response strategies. Disaster response includes basic elements that are similar in all events. The difference is the degree to which these elements are utilized in a specific incident, and the degree to which outside assistance is needed. The National Incident Management System (NIMS) is designed to standardize this response across the nation to provide consistent incident management.[6]

First responders at the scene must attempt to establish command and control, regardless of the size, nature, or complexity of the scene, and regardless of their experience level. Of course, safety remains the top priority—personal safety followed by that of the response team. To coordinate response efforts, the overall command and control function can and should be transferred to more senior or expert personnel, as response agencies formulate an incident command system at the scene.

6.6.1   Incident Command

The concept of the incident command system (ICS) was developed in the aftermath of 13 days of devastating wildfires in California in 1970. Many factors contributed to this disaster, including:

➤ A lack of common organization

➤ Poor on-scene and interagency communications

➤ Inadequate resource management

➤ Limited prediction capability

➤ Use of different operational procedures and terminology and incompatible equipment

➤ Overlap of governmental jurisdictions

As a result, Congress mandated that the US Forest Service design a system that would "make a quantum jump in the capabilities of Southern California wildland fire protection agencies to effectively coordinate interagency action and to allocate suppression resources in dynamic, multiple-fire situations." The resulting working group, and the body of work they developed, known collectively as FIRESCOPE (FIrefighting RESources of California Organized for Potential Emergencies), serve as the root of what we today know as the incident command system.[7]

The ICS has become the model for disaster management needs throughout the nation. The current challenge is to maximize the use of ICS, across geographic and disciplinary borders, so that this proven approach can be applied to incident management needs nationwide. Figure 6-1 illustrates the structure of the ICS.

Application of the ICS is dynamic. It may be expanded or scaled down depending on the:

➤ Type of incident

➤ Changes that may occur during operation

➤ Number of casualties

➤ Available resources

The ICS is based on the following overarching concepts:

➤ *Unity of command.* At any disaster scene, there is a single designated supervisor, referred to as the incident commander. The incident commander is ultimately responsible for the overall management of the situation. This person employs the expertise and wisdom of a command staff composed of a public information officer, a safety officer, and a liaison officer. Additionally, the incident commander and his or her command staff rely on

FIGURE 6-1
Structure of the ICS

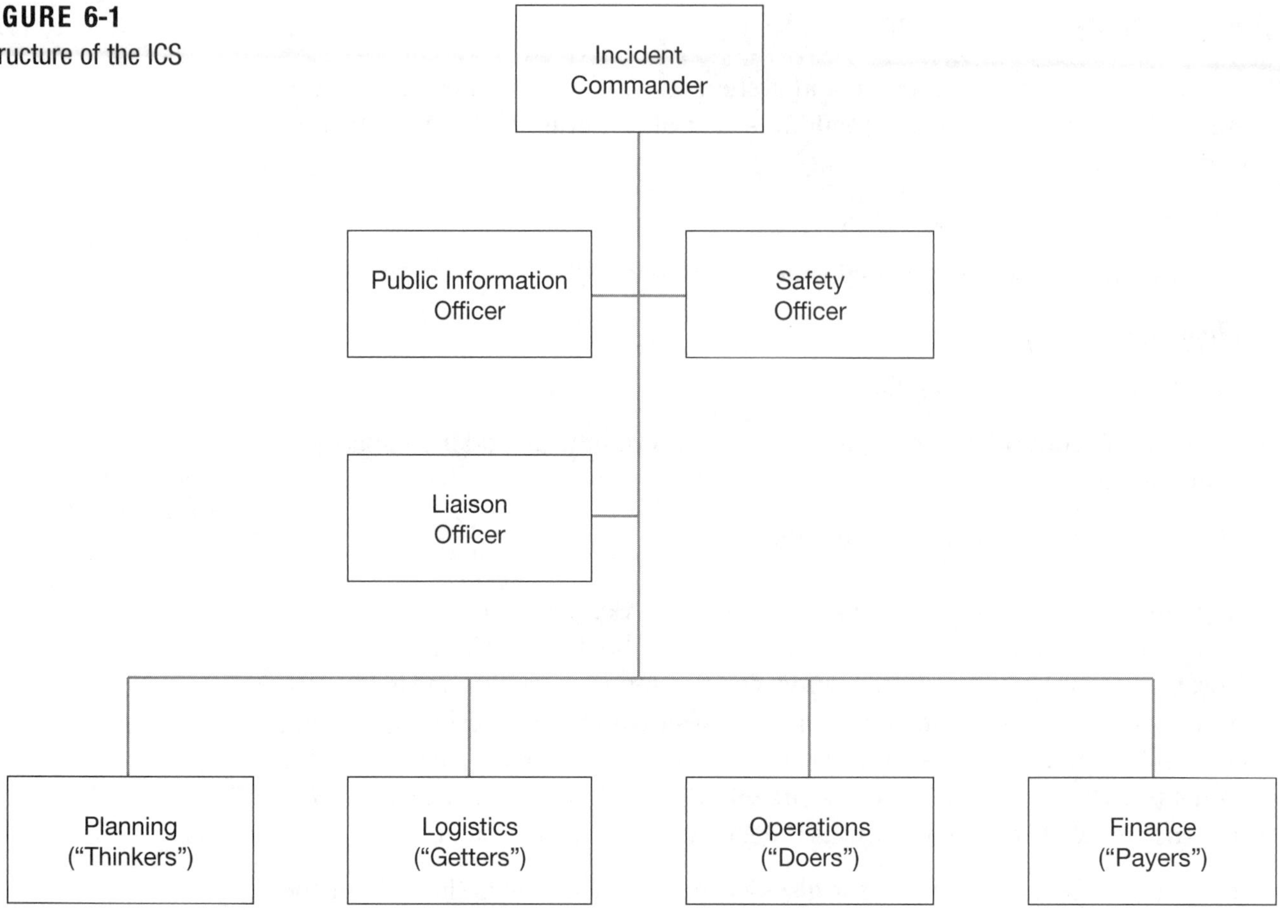

```
                        ┌──────────────┐
                        │   Incident   │
                        │  Commander   │
                        └──────┬───────┘
                               │
          ┌──────────────┐     │     ┌──────────────┐
          │    Public    │     │     │    Safety    │
          │  Information ├─────┼─────┤   Officer    │
          │   Officer    │     │     │              │
          └──────────────┘     │     └──────────────┘
                               │
          ┌──────────────┐     │
          │   Liaison    ├─────┤
          │   Officer    │     │
          └──────────────┘     │
                               │
    ┌──────────┬───────────────┼───────────────┬──────────┐
┌───┴────┐ ┌───┴────┐     ┌────┴─────┐     ┌────┴────┐
│Planning│ │Logistics│    │Operations│     │ Finance │
│("Think-│ │("Getters")│  │("Doers") │     │("Payers")│
│ ers")  │ │         │    │          │     │         │
└────────┘ └─────────┘    └──────────┘     └─────────┘
```

a general staff to supervise the four major functional elements of the ICS. These are the operations section, planning section, logistics section, and finance/administration section.

In most cases, health professionals will not serve as incident commanders. This role is best left to fire and law enforcement personnel with specific training and experience with the ICS. However, in the case of a public health emergency, such as an infectious disease outbreak, the public health director may be the incident commander. The incident commander may not be the person who normally leads an organization on a daily basis, and may or may not be an expert in the particular type of disaster, but must be a capable manager and leader. In the case of hospitals, each hospital will establish its own ICS or similar system. The most commonly used is the Hospital Incident Command System (HICS). Under HICS the commander is designated in advance of the incident.

➤ *Orderly line of authority.* Officers direct personnel within their respective sections and report back to the incident commander. This line of authority means that every person working in each section knows his or her role and to whom he or she reports. Incident command sections must work in harmony among themselves and with the incident commander at all times. They must maintain control of resources and facilitate communication both up and down the organizational structure.

➤ *Span of control.* An important component of an ICS is a manageable span of control. The *span of control* refers to the number of individuals who are reporting to any one individual. A tight span of control is important for the flow of information, resource allotment, and overall operations response. A good ICS setup limits the number of individuals reporting to any leader to no more than 7 and preferably only 5.

➤ *Standardized and scalable response.* ICS principles can be applied to any size or type of event by any size of agency. A scalable response indicates that the response can be smaller or larger, depending on the scope and magnitude of the event. A common understanding and terminology are extremely important in incident command. This reduces confusion about responder roles during a disaster.

6.6.2   Incident Command Structures

Incident command typically involves a single agency as the primary responder. If there are multiple agencies involved, the situation requires use of unified command or area command structures. For most emergencies, the ICS will be composed of a network of professionals, working on common goals, under the leadership of one ultimately responsible commander.

Single Incident Command.   This ICS structure is used for smaller events, such as a house fire, involving a single response agency. While this level of incident may still require some or all ICS components, in this case, the highest-ranking fire officer on the scene would be the incident commander.

Unified Incident Command.   This ICS structure is used in situations in which more than one responding agency has responsibility for the incident, and/or when the incident involves multiple jurisdictions. These jurisdictions could be represented by:

➤ Geographic boundaries (cities, states, tribal land)

➤ Governmental levels (local, state, federal)

➤ Functional responsibilities (such as firefighting, EMS, and law enforcement)

➤ Some combination of the above

While the vast majority of incidents are resolved by using the single command structure, large-scale emergencies may require that the ICS be expanded to a unified command structure. This structure brings together the incident commanders of all major organizations involved in the incident in an effort to coordinate an effective response while at the same time carrying out their own jurisdictional responsibilities. Unified command links all organizations responding to the incident and provides a forum for the leaders of these entities to make fully informed, consensus decisions that allow their respective agencies to work together to resolve the situation.

Under unified command, the various jurisdictions and/or agencies and nongovernment responders work together in a single, centralized command post for coordinating and supporting incident management activities. These resources may include facilities, equipment, personnel, procedures, and communications. The primary functions of multiagency coordination are to:

➤ Support and coordinate incident management among participating agencies

➤ Facilitate logistics support and resource tracking and information

➤ Make resource allocation decisions on the basis of incident priorities

In a unified command structure, the role of the incident commander is commonly filled by fire or law enforcement (local or Federal Bureau of Investigation) personnel, depending on the type of incident. The incident commander oversees incident management, sets goals and priorities, and delegates the management of the planning, logistics, operations, and finance sections (refer to Figure 6-1).

➤ *Planning Section ("The Thinkers"):* These personnel collect, evaluate, and disseminate information to and from the scene. The group maintains resource inventory and incident-related documentation and records a log of the incident. The members review existing plans designed to guide a response to the incident at hand. They also formulate plans for the hours, days, and weeks ahead for responding to the event.

➤ *Logistics Section ("The Getters"):* These personnel are responsible for identifying and providing services and support. This includes communications, transportation, fuel, and personnel needs such as food, sanitation, shelter, water, and health services.

➤ *Operations Section ("The Doers"):* These personnel oversee the operations or activities at the scene of an event or in the hospital to accomplish the mission of responding to the disaster event. In a disaster, health professionals are most likely to participate as part of the operations section and are responsible for rendering care to the victims. Rescue and fire operations may involve helping trapped or stranded people or deploying personnel to fight the fire. The operations section may be divided into several sectors on the basis of their respective missions (eg, health, fire, rescue, etc).

➤ *Finance Section ("The Payers").* These personnel assess and track incident-related costs, maintain personnel and equipment records, and administer any contracting needs.

Area Command. This ICS structure is used for event coordination when there is no incident scene. It includes standard ICS organization except for the operations section. In an area command, an incident commander is still responsible for incident management activities. Depending on the complexity of the incident and span-of-control considerations, an area command is established to oversee one of two situations:

➤ The management of multiple incidents that are being handled by separate ICS organizations or

➤ The management of a very large incident that involves multiple ICS organizations

Response to a large-scale infectious disease outbreak may require an area command structure, involving multiple jurisdictions and agencies, to determine responsibilities and coordinate the allocation of potentially scarce health resources.

6.6.3   Hospital Incident Command System

The ICS also applies to hospitals and other health care facilities. The Joint Commission requires all hospitals to utilize a command system that follows the principles and objectives of the ICS for dealing with both internal and external

---

Incident Management Training for Health Care Professionals and Other Responders

The FEMA Emergency Management Institute provides numerous educational and training opportunities on incident management through classroom-based and online courses. Courses and curricula have been developed collaboratively with the US Department of Homeland Security (DHS), the National Wildfire Coordinating Group, the US Fire Administration, and the US Department of Agriculture. The DHS recommends that all key personnel involved in community and facility emergency management and incident response take the following National Incident Management System (NIMS)–compliant independent study courses as applicable:

➤ IS-100.a (ICS 100), Introduction to Incident Command System

➤ IS-100.HC, Introduction to the Incident Command System for Healthcare/Hospitals

➤ IS-100.HE, Introduction to the Incident Command System for Higher Education

➤ IS-100.LEa, Introduction to the Incident Command System for Law Enforcement

➤ IS-100.PWa, Introduction to the Incident Command System for Public Works Personnel

➤ IS-100.SCa, Introduction to the Incident Command System for Schools

➤ IS-200.HC, Applying ICS to Healthcare Organizations

➤ IS-700.a, National Incident Management System (NIMS), an Introduction

➤ IS-800.b, National Response Framework (NRF), an Introduction

More information about the Emergency Management Institute and its training program is available at http://training.fema.gov/.

disasters. The Hospital Incident Command System (HICS), which was created in the late 1980s by the California EMS Authority as an important foundation in preparing for emergencies and is used by many hospitals and health care agencies throughout the country.[8] As with incident command in the field, the HICS provides common terminology to enhance communication and improve documentation. Duties are assigned by position and include a clear chain of authority and command. Health care workers must know their specific facility command structure and how they fit into its chain of command.

6.6.4   Emergency Operations Center

The emergency operations center (EOC) is a central command and control location responsible for carrying out the principles of emergency management at a strategic level in an emergency. An EOC is the location for coordination of information and resources to support incident activities. It facilitates the safe, effective operation of the ICS at the scene and ensures the continuity of operations for the affected region during and after the disaster. An EOC is the physical location where the leaders of a region or organization come together during an emergency or disaster to analyze response and recovery options, coordinate actions, and allocate resources. These centers may alternatively be called *crisis management centers*, *command centers*, *situation rooms*, *war rooms*, or the like.

The EOC is not an incident command post; rather, it is the operations center where coordination and management decisions are facilitated, decisions that in many instances equip the incident commander with the tools needed to get the job done at the scene. In a public health emergency, it is likely that a health EOC will be established to help coordinate medical and public health response efforts. Standing up an EOC focused solely on health can be an integral component of the response and is necessary to maximize the health care response to the event.

6.7   SAFETY/SECURITY AND ASSESS HAZARDS

The nature of emergency response is to save lives, which may involve responders putting their own safety at risk. If the precise cause of an incident is not immediately apparent, or if there is a suspicion that something is unusual, emergency responders should take necessary precautions to minimize risk to themselves and others. Even if real-time identification of the precise cause is possible, responder safety remains paramount. Triage, treatment, and evacuation of casualties become secondary considerations if scene conditions do not permit intervention without endangering rescuers. The immediate scene may be too dangerous to allow any responders in to provide care.

6.7.1   Scene Priorities

During a disaster, everyone on the scene—including first responders and volunteers—is responsible for scene safety and security. This includes being familiar with basic scene priorities and specific considerations for various hazards that may be encountered.

Regardless of the cause of the disaster, safety is the top priority at any incident scene. Safety involves protecting oneself, protecting others at the scene, and protecting the community and the environment.

Protecting Oneself.   When confronted with a disaster, the first priority should be protection of personal safety. It should be remembered that a person will contribute little to disaster response if he or she becomes a casualty. If responders are injured or killed, not only can they not help anyone else, but they have increased the casualty load and decreased the response capacity of their team. Safe response begins with sound mental preparation. Responders should mentally run through potential realistic scenarios. How could each situation most safely and effectively be handled? Visualization can be an effective tool that can help responders prepare for a situation and feel as if they have been there before, creating a sense of readiness and capability. In many instances, just getting to the scene safely can be a challenge. It is important to have planned response routes and to be constantly vigilant of potential dangers.

Protecting Others at the Scene.   After ensuring personal safety, it is necessary to consider how to protect other responders and bystanders from injury, as well to prevent further harm to those who need assistance. Responders should protect the scene by preventing bystanders or other untrained persons from entering the area. Responders may be able to help protect injured persons by assisting with their evacuation to a safe area.

Protecting the Community and the Environment.   Protecting the general public and the environment can be best accomplished by communicating with appropriate local and state officials.

6.7.2   Hazard Assessment

A challenging feature of many disasters is the risk of structural collapse, fire, ruptured gas lines, downed power lines, and numerous other factors, which may trigger additional casualties. Other concerns can include the potential release of toxic chemicals and radiation, as well as respiratory hazards from byproducts of combustion (eg, smoke, carbon monoxide, cyanide, or dust). Emergency responders must take appropriate precautions to protect themselves and others. If they do not, detection of these situations may come too late to prevent further harm and destruction.

The "Dos" and "Don'ts" of Scene Safety and Security

DO:

➤ Protect self and others from harm

➤ Communicate potential hazards to others

➤ Communicate effectively with the appropriate chain of command of emergency services/emergency management personnel

➤ Enforce restricted access as directed or advised by incident command

➤ Always proceed as though the scene may be contaminated

➤ Remain vigilant for secondary hazards

DON'T:

➤ Don't show up unless requested/dispatched. While a responder's skills may be needed, especially during a large disaster, they will be utilized at the request of the incident commander or his or her designee. Responders should notify emergency personnel of skills and abide by their commands

➤ Don't enter the scene without adequate protection. The scene environment should be considered unsafe, uncertain, and unpredictable

➤ Don't become another casualty

➤ Don't contribute to a traffic problems, which could delay rescue. Access routes may be limited

➤ Don't disturb the scene. A disaster scene may be a crime scene, and everything could be evidence

All disasters, regardless of the primary cause, create the possibility of secondary hazards capable of injuring anyone present at the scene, including responders. The detonation of a car bomb, for example, can be more than just a simple explosion. The bomb also may be associated with the release of a chemical or radioactive agent. A secondary device may be left behind at the scene to explode when the device is moved or touched by response personnel. The explosion can cause additional damage to surrounding buildings and infrastructure. Incident response can be further complicated by communications disruption; weather threats; loss of routes of ingress and egress; damage to emergency vehicles, equipment, and supplies; and even darkness. The all-hazards approach to disaster response requires awareness of the possibility of such dangers and continual assessment at the scene to detect and protect against recognized and perceived threats.

In any mass casualty incident, many people can be expected to self-transport to the nearest hospitals. In most large-scale disasters, 70% to 80% of victims will self-transport. Self-transport means that they will get there by private or public transportation, without EMS involvement or decontamination. It is critical to consider the potential risk that such persons present at hospitals and other receiving facilities, not to mention the potential for contamination of vehicles and other persons en route.

In most HAZMAT cases, the command post should be located outdoors, upwind, upstream, and/or uphill from the scene to minimize exposure to airborne hazards. Most chemical agents create vapors that are denser than air and that tend to settle in low-lying areas. Therefore, the scene should be immediately evacuated uphill and upwind from the release site. Chemicals can induce symptoms quickly, so immediate action should be taken for casualty evacuation and decontamination. Precautions must be taken to protect personnel from contamination.

A biologic event presents a difficult challenge because there may not be a "disaster scene," or the mode of release may be very difficult to detect. This means that discovery of the event may be delayed. Sick people will go to physician offices, clinics, and emergency departments over a period of time, exposing others to the disease.

6.7.3 Risk Reduction Measures

Risk reduction measures are implemented to lower the possibility of exposure to actual or potential hazards. For disaster responders, this involves administrative controls (eg, respiratory protection programs, disaster plans, standard operating procedures), engineering controls (eg, shut-down of heating and air conditioning systems, sprinkler systems, negative–air pressure rooms in hospitals), the use of personal protective equipment (PPE), and decontamination. Engineering controls are used to remove a hazard at the scene, to remove reliance on human behavior, or to place a barrier between responders and the hazard. Well-designed engineering controls can be highly effective in protecting responders. When engineering solutions are not feasible, administrative controls offer methods to reduce exposure. Administrative controls are policies, procedures, and practices that minimize the exposure of responders and affected populations to hazardous conditions. They are considered less effective than engineering controls in that they do not usually eliminate the hazard and they rely on human behavior.

Possible Hazards at a Disaster Scene

It is important to remember that scene safety is a dynamic concept. While it is critically important to ensure a safe scene prior to entry, it is equally important to stay attuned to changes that take place at the disaster scene as the situation develops. Examples include, but are not limited to:

- Animals and insects
- Blood and body fluid exposure
- Communication disruption
- Contamination of air, food, and water
- Darkness
- Debris
- Downed power lines
- Environmental exposure (heat, cold)
- Equipment-related injuries (chain saws)
- Explosions
- Fire
- Flooding
- Hazardous materials release (chemical, biologic, radiologic)
- Motor vehicle crashes
- Ruptured gas lines
- Secondary explosive devices
- Smoke and toxic gases (eg, carbon monoxide)
- Snipers/gunman
- Structural collapse

Rather, they lessen the duration and frequency of exposure to the situation. The least effective controls are PPE and decontamination, as responders are still present in a hazardous environment.

Personal Protective Equipment.   The purpose of PPE is to minimize contact with contaminated persons, objects, or scenes.[9] This includes protecting the skin, mouth, eyes, nose, lungs, and other body parts vulnerable to vapor or liquid exposure and penetration. PPE includes two components: (1) respiratory protection and (2) protective garments and barriers.

PPE is a critical component of scene safety, regardless of the disaster; it provides a hazard barrier that allows function in a hazardous area and must be used properly during all phases of response. Some level of PPE will be needed before entering any disaster scene. Casualty care may have to wait until proper PPE is available. Proper selection of the appropriate level of protection (A, B, C, D, or Bio-PPE) will depend on the unique circumstances of the event. It should be noted that PPE may refer to hazardous-materials PPE.

➤ *Level A PPE* should be worn when the highest level of respiratory, skin, eye, and mucous membrane protection is needed. It consists of a fully encapsulated, vapor-tight, chemical-resistant suit with a self-contained breathing apparatus or positive-pressure air line, and chemical-resistant boots and gloves. The rescuer cannot don or remove this suit without assistance, and any movement while in the suit is severely restricted. Many personnel find performing the simplest of tasks difficult while in level A PPE. It is used primarily by trained HAZMAT personnel in a heavily contaminated environment. Proper use of level A PPE requires previous training, fitting, and experience. The sight of personnel on scene working in this level of protection should be a signal to evacuate immediately to a safer location.

➤ *Level B PPE* should be worn when the highest level of respiratory protection is needed, but a lesser degree of skin protection is required. It differs from level A in that it provides splash protection only through the use of chemical-resistant clothing, face protection, boots, and gloves with a self-contained breathing apparatus or positive-pressure air line. The user can be tethered to a hose connected to a remote air source or to a supplied-air respirator. Level B PPE also includes a hooded chemical-resistant suit and includes face protection, boots, and gloves. Proper use requires previous training, fitting, and experience. The sight of personnel at the scene in level B PPE connotes a heavily contaminated scene and demands immediate evacuation to a safer location.

➤ *Level C PPE* provides limited respiratory protection in that it filters the ambient air. It includes an air-purifying respirator, not a supplied air source.

The respirator can be a powered air-purifying respirator or nonpowered device that uses the wearer's ability to pull air through filters located on the mask. Level C consists of a hooded chemical-resistant suit, along with boots and gloves.

➤ *Level D PPE* provides the minimum protection against contamination and provides no respiratory protection. Level D consists of standard work uniforms or work clothes. In a hospital environment, the blood-borne pathogens protection (also called "universal precautions") typically used provides appropriate level D protection. This includes a fluid impermeable gown, cap, eye protection, mask, gloves, and shoes. This level of protection is suitable for noncontaminated patients and for patients with radioactive contamination.

➤ *Bio-PPE* entails the use of standard work clothes along with contact and respiratory protection. This includes double gloves, impermeable gowns, goggles, cap, leg and shoe covers, and an N95 mask (or better) respirator. Hand hygiene consisting of washing with soap or use of alcohol gel is very important. When compared to the other PPE levels, bio-PPE falls between level C and level D protection. It is sufficient for protection against radio-active materials and biologic agents in the hospital setting after patient decontamination. Bio-PPE is not sufficient before decontamination, or for use at or near a hazardous materials release site.

No single PPE combination protects against every possible hazard. In addition, certain types of PPE create risks for the wearer. The proper use and limitations of PPE are discussed more in the BDLS and ADLS courses.

Decontamination. A disaster involving a chemical agent or radioactive material may create the need for decontamination. In this case, no one should enter the scene or approach injured persons without appropriate PPE. If contaminated patients arrive at a health care facility, they should not be allowed to enter the facility until decontaminated.

Decontamination is a primary objective for initial casualty care. The decision to decontaminate should be made early, even if it is based on incomplete information. Once the decision is made to proceed, it should be assumed that every exposed individual is contaminated until proven otherwise. In some instances, such as after nerve agent or cyanide exposure, antidote administration must proceed simultaneously with or prior to decontamination by health care providers in PPE.

Decontamination is generally performed by trained and appropriately equipped personnel to reduce a person's exposure to hazardous materials and minimize the chance of secondary contamination of responders, health care providers, and others. It involves the process of removing or deactivating harmful contaminants from external body surfaces. The two basic types of decontamination are "dry" and "wet." Dry decontamination is acceptable when there is a vapor exposure only. If contact has occurred on the skin, wet decontamination must occur.

➤ *Dry decontamination* includes removal of all clothing, shoes, socks, undergarments, jewelry, and contact lenses. It can also include self-cleaning with a cloth or other supplied material.

➤ *Wet decontamination* includes the steps of dry decontamination, plus a low-volume wash with soap and water or water-based solution, scrubbing of external body surfaces, and use of specific neutralizing or deactivating substances. Wet decontamination may be performed on ambulatory (walking) persons or on casualties transported on stretchers.

Because many people self-transport from large mass casualty incidents, it should be expected that contaminated patients will arrive at health care facilities after an incident involving chemical or radiologic hazards. Hospital decontamination can be performed by setting up portable decontamination tents or by modifying existing facility infrastructure to create spaces that can rapidly be converted to a mass decontamination facility. Parking garages, for example, can be modified by installing curtains, heaters, and shower heads to create large decontamination facilities capable of handling hundreds of patients per hour. Mutual aid resources, such as local fire departments, also may be useful because they have experience in decontamination and are familiar with decontamination equipment. However, these resources may not be immediately available and may be in demand by multiple facilities, and therefore health care facilities should not rely on their availability during an event.

All persons who are decontaminated will require temporary clothing and blankets appropriate for the climate. Once decontamination is completed, provisions must be made for additional medical and mental health care. Patients should receive a medical screening examination to determine the need for further care. Those who do not require definitive treatment can be moved to a separate area for observation and monitoring for delayed symptoms. Those requiring medical attention should be triaged and transported to the appropriate care area.

Biosafety and Infection Control Precautions.

Careful attention must be given to persons who are suspected of having been exposed to or infected with an infectious biologic agent. Some biologic agents are easily transmitted from person to person and may require isolation or quarantine. Disease transmission risks also mandate the use of appropriate PPE for emergency and health personnel. Public health authorities should be alerted as soon as possible for guidance and assistance.

Knowledge of biosafety and infection control procedures and observance of established protocols are important for all disaster responders. With the litany of disease and infection possibilities that exist, particularly those involving a serious communicable disease agent, adhering to universal precautions, while seemingly basic, can be a critical step in limiting disease transmission. As a general rule, responders and health care providers should consider the need for PPE when presented with any patient with a fever and a cough.

6.8 SUPPORT

By its very nature, a disaster or serious mass casualty incident requires the coordination of resources and assets from myriad public and private sector agencies and organizations. As described in Chapter 3, effective response, recovery, and mitigation require support planning by agencies, institutions, and communities well in advance of any emergency. Successful mitigation and management of any event begins with thorough and detailed planning, drills, analysis of information collected from drills, and historical information from actual disaster events. Planning and "what if" scenarios are integral components to successful support preparedness, as well as successful event mitigation.

Disaster support encompasses a spectrum of resources, including human resources, agencies, facilities, supplies, and vehicles. As described in Chapter 4, a wide range of support services and agencies is available, from local volunteers to large federal programs. Some are available to assist in the early hours of disaster response. Others, such as the National Disaster Medical System (NDMS) teams, provide backup for depleted personnel and resources in the days after an event.[10] The Strategic National Stockpile provides a national repository of emergency pharmaceuticals, medical supplies, and equipment that can be shipped anywhere in the United States in response to a national emergency.[11] The infrastructure for providing support under normal, day-to-day emergencies already exists in most communities; through mutual aid, the resources in a neighboring community can be brought into the affected areas to provide additional assistance. The Chem-Pak program administered by the CDC is a regional stockpile program that locates time-sensitive antidotes and antibiotics in the communities to speed the response. State-sponsored disaster teams can often respond faster than the federal system, but these assets vary widely from state to state. In a disaster, the response time, type, and amount of support needed can fluctuate significantly.

NIMS recognizes the need for additional support as a staple in all disaster situations and provides steps to make gathering that support more efficient. This includes the development of a system wherein personnel are uniformly credentialed and included in a database such as Emergency System for Advance Registration of Volunteer Health Professionals (ESAR-VHP), and where equipment is similarly cataloged and identified in a resource management process. Like the ICS, under NIMS, resource management is flexible and scalable to be able to meet the dynamic needs of any disaster scene.

The nature, size, and scope of a disaster, and the scene it creates, will dictate the prioritization of available resources and response assets to meet the needs of affected populations. Every emergency and every disaster is unique in this regard. Effective disaster management hinges on the timely delivery of resources to where they are needed most. Support may not be given much thought until resources are depleted, by which time its arrival may be too late to help change the outcome.

6.8.1   Human Resources

Human resource activation and management is critical. This entails an accurate assessment of the number of responders and the skills required, as well as the means to ensure that they are available and willing to respond. There must be sufficient resources to replace tired or injured responders and to activate other responders as demands evolve.

Human resources that must be considered during response consist of not only various levels of health professionals, but also firefighters, law enforcement personnel, bomb squad, heavy rescue and HAZMAT teams, construction workers, equipment operators, warehouse personnel, truck drivers, administrators, financial and accounting personnel, photographers, and housekeeping staff, to name a few. In addition, human resource needs may exist that are unique to a specific disaster, such as events requiring decontamination, criminal investigation, or mass fatality management.

6.8.2   Agencies

As described in Chapter 4, many types of public and private sector agencies and organizations are capable of providing support during a disaster. These agencies may be local organizations unique to a specific community, such as outreach organizations, places of worship, and clubs. The American Red Cross, Salvation Army, and other nongovernmental organizations are valuable assets that provide support during a disaster.

6.8.3   Facilities

Facilities required for the management of a disaster will depend on the type of event. For example, if the situation requires decontamination of casualties, then decontamination facilities may be required both at the scene and at receiving facilities such as hospitals. To provide for the basic health care needs for the community, alternate care locations may be required at various venues throughout the community. These sites may reduce the demand and risk to persons transported directly from the scene to area hospitals.

Other facility considerations in a disaster may include the need for shelter, food, clothing, and housing for affected populations. This requirement also must be considered for the responders, staff, and volunteers involved in event mitigation. Warehouse space may be required for the receipt and distribution of supplies; for volunteer reporting, work assignments, and transport; and for equipment maintenance and repair.

6.8.4   Supplies

Items such as food, water, shelter, heaters, blankets, cots, medical supplies, rescue tools and equipment, batteries, generators, and fuel will be needed in quantities commensurate with the extent of the disaster. Health care supplies for medical support can largely be categorized as pharmaceuticals or consumables. Pharmaceutical supplies must be properly controlled, accounted for, and stored. The Strategic National Stockpile requires extensive planning for its receipt, storage, and distribution. Supplies for the first 24 hours are limited largely to those available locally unless regional or state stockpiles are kept as well.

Complete mobilization of requested supplies from outside sources will take hours to days or weeks. When the outside supplies arrive, facilities, human resources, and equipment must be provided for receipt, stocking, packaging, and distribution. These processes can cause further delays.

6.8.5   Vehicles

Vehicle considerations during hazardous incidents include the provision of EMS, fire department, and law enforcement response vehicles, and fixed-wing aircraft or helicopters. In addition, buses and shuttles, pickups, tractor-trailer rigs, boats, heavy equipment (earthmovers and bulldozers), cranes and trucks, and the personnel to operate them may be necessary to respond to the event.

6.8.6   Medical Support and Surge Capacity[12,13]

Immediately after a disaster, injured but ambulatory persons will largely evacuate themselves and proceed to the nearest health care facility. Layperson rescuers also will take injured persons to the nearest health care facility, regardless of the seriousness of the injury. This response can overload health care facilities in the first 30 to 60 minutes after the event. Such overloading may not only exhaust resources at the facility, but also may shut it down altogether because of contamination or other problems. Procedures to obtain additional capacity during a disaster must be both preestablished and flexible, with predetermined methods of activating these resources for different levels of response.

Surge capacity refers to the ability of the health care facility to care for a mark-edly increased volume of patients.[14] *Surge capability* refers to caring for patients who require unusual or very specialized care or evaluation.[14]

During a disaster, hospital staff will have to deal with an influx of persons who need or think they need prompt attention. A challenge then becomes how to meet their demands while continuing to meet the needs of patients who were already receiving care in the facility before the event and the potential additional medical/trauma needs, unrelated to the event, that may present in the coming hours. The success of meeting these challenges lies in a number of variables, not the least of which is location of the facility. In an urban or suburban hospital the impact of the disaster may be dissipated across multiple facilities, thus blunting the impact on any one facility. In the setting of a rural hospital, there may be no additional hospital to absorb the impact of the event. Rural facilities can succeed as well but must plan for how they will react, perhaps by involving neighboring counties or communities to provide relief.

Establishing surge capacity to meet increased health-related needs in a disaster consists of three primary medical support areas: human resources, facilities, and supplies. The availability of these resources is limited by the routine needs of a community and by the economics and logistics involved in creating and main-taining excess capacity from normal community requirements in a serious mass casualty event. A disaster in no way reduces the demand for "normal" baseline community health care. Asthma, dialysis, surgery, cardiac events, trauma, child-birth, and other conditions still need to be addressed and must be considered.

Patient bed availability in hospitals becomes a critical factor during a mass casualty event, especially for those hospitals in proximity to the disaster scene. Additional patient bed capacity might be obtained by moving or discharging existing patients to other more distant facilities, and by transporting the "well but worried" or "walking wounded" to secondary facilities, facilities outside the com-munity, urgent care centers, or other locations. Secondary or field hospitals can be set up and distributed throughout a community to alleviate high concentrations of patients in one area. While this process could increase patient bed capacity, it would also increase the need for various supplies and human resources (such as drivers, EMS personnel, nurses, doctors, and facility administrators).

Local mortuary capacity also may be exceeded in a very short period of time. Depending on the size and type of the event, additional mortuary capacity may be needed immediately. Alternatives might include local funeral homes; appropriate facilities that can be utilized temporarily as morgues (large coolers); refrigerated trucks for transporting fatalities to more distant morgues; or on-site mortuary facilities or secondary temporary facilities established for this purpose.

Laboratory capacity may be limited during a disaster. For routine laboratory requirements, special couriers and transport systems can be established to dis-tribute the demand over larger geographic areas. Laboratory tests should be limited to those necessary for diagnosis and treatment of more critically ill or injured patients. Some specific tests may be postponed to a more appropriate and less demanding time. For laboratory tests requiring specialized laboratory equipment or capabilities, samples may require transport to regional, state, or federal laboratory sites. Arrangements for testing require prior communication and arrangements.

6.9 TRIAGE AND TREATMENT

All disasters, regardless of cause, have some similarities in their medical and public health consequences. The events differ in the degree to which these consequences occur and the degree to which they disrupt the medical and public health infrastructure in the affected region. When disaster strikes, emergency needs at the scene may quickly overwhelm local resources. Mass casualty incidents can quickly exceed the resources of local health care facilities, particularly when numerous people are injured simultaneously with life-threatening, multiorgan injuries. Access to medical resources may be limited by communication, transportation, and other constraints. To save the most lives possible, quick decisions must be made for the efficient use of immediately available resources. To accomplish this, emergency responders rely on triage systems.

In day-to-day emergencies, a triage situation requires the temporary prioritization of medical care delivered in physician offices, clinics, and emergency departments, with the objective to do the greatest good for each individual patient. In a serious disaster, involving multiple casualties, this objective changes to doing the greatest good for the greatest number of possible survivors. It is essential to remember this distinction during any serious disaster or public health emergency. The initial goal of disaster triage is to sort casualties to identify those with life threatening injuries in order to initiate life-saving treatment immediately. Once this is accomplished, casualties with less serious injuries can be assessed further and triaged for transportation from the scene on the basis of their level of injury and available resources.

6.9.1 Mass Casualty Triage

Triage may be defined as the sorting of people by the seriousness of their condition and by the likelihood of their survival and is one of the most important missions of any disaster health response. Decisions made during triage have an important impact on the health outcomes of affected individuals and communities. Disaster triage involves rapid categorization of casualties with potentially severe injuries who require immediate medical attention at the scene. In a disaster, health care needs exceed the immediately available resources, and therefore, not all casualties may receive full medical care. In a serious mass casualty event, this can be a daunting and difficult challenge.

Field triage will most likely be performed by first responders from the local population or local emergency response personnel. Ideally, casualties will be rapidly categorized at a designated triage site at the scene by the most experienced medical personnel available to identify the level of care that is needed. Knowledge of the basic medical consequences of various injuries (eg, burn, blast, or crush injuries or exposure to chemical, biologic, and radioactive agents) is critical. Knowledge of such consequences in children is particularly important.[15] However, the initial steps of triage may be performed by the bystanders on the scene and requires little more than a basic understanding of the process.

The challenge faced by responders in a serious mass casualty event is that not all affected persons, injured or otherwise, can be attended to at once. A systematic method is needed to quickly determine which people need treatment most urgently. The immediate goal is to help as many injured persons as possible with the resources available at a given moment in time. For many responders, this presents a difficult dilemma because it is only natural to want to help everyone who is injured. The challenge lies in remaining calm and remembering that there may be casualties that require urgent lifesaving intervention. In the first few moments of triage in a mass casualty event, responders need to adhere to a uniform system, which is designed to help them find the most critically injured persons who may survive if stabilized at the scene and transported with priority to an area hospital for more definitive medical care.

6.9.2 Triage Systems

In a disaster, there may be many casualties and only a few responders. There may be little or no time for intensive one-on-one assessment and care. An efficient system is needed to rapidly identify casualties most in need of—and most likely to benefit from—immediate care.

There are several different mass casualty triage systems in use, derived from both military and civilian sources.[16-19] These systems may employ different methods of classifying and tagging casualties by using symbols, colors, and other conventions. Health care workers, first responders, and EMS personnel should become familiar with the triage system used by their organization or agency and work to standardize the systems used across all components of the disaster response system. To minimize confusion and maximize communication, it would be ideal if all responders—field personnel and hospital personnel—used the same triage system.

Recently, a proposed national standard for mass casualty triage was developed through a collaborative effort funded by the CDC.[16, 20] The system is called *SALT*, which stands for *S*ort, *A*ssess, *L*ifesaving interventions, and *T*reatment and/or transport. SALT is a simple mnemonic that is easy to remember. It was developed to facilitate the management of large numbers of casualties quickly to determine whether there are lifesaving interventions that need to be administered.

Step 1. In the first step in SALT, the sorting process, casualties are prioritized for more individualized assessment through simple voice commands, like asking them to walk to a designated area or wave their hands. Other triage systems usually sort patients by asking them to walk but then consider those persons to be minimally injured without conducting further individual assessment. This might cause some people who are able to walk but need immediate care to be ignored for extended periods of time. In SALT triage, the ability to walk indicates that persons most likely have:

➤ Airway, breathing, and circulation intact (these persons are not likely to have low blood pressure or breathing problems); and

➤ Mental status intact, at least to the extent that they can follow simple commands.

The SALT triage method requires that these persons be individually assessed at some point to determine the extent of any injuries, but this initial step of triage can be performed by a disaster responder or bystander.

Simple voice commands are used to prioritize patients for individual assessment and to give those who can walk clear instructions regarding where to go for help. These instructions may keep people from self-triaging to the closest hospital by giving them a specific place to go for additional assistance. The "wave" command allows responders to distinguish persons who are not able to follow a command from those who can follow a command but cannot walk; this gives responders an opportunity to more easily identify which injured people need critical care. By assessing those persons who are not waving or making purposeful movements first, triage personnel are more likely to approach those injured persons who may require urgent lifesaving intervention.

The second step of SALT triage should only be performed by those persons with more formal training in mass casualty triage and medical care. It is presented here to introduce the concept to those learners who have or will pursue more advanced training.

Step 2. During step 2 of SALT triage, remaining casualties are assessed individually, sorted into initial triage categories, and transported from the scene as appropriate. The first priority during this assessment is to provide lifesaving interventions. These include controlling major hemorrhage, opening the airway, chest needle decompression for persons with tension pneumothorax, and providing autoinjector antidotes for chemical exposures. These interventions were selected because they can be applied rapidly and can have a considerable impact on survival.

Once lifesaving interventions have been provided, casualties are prioritized for treatment on the basis of assignment to one of five categories.: *immediate, delayed, minimal, expectant,* and *dead.* A simple mnemonic, ID-MED, can be used to remember these triage categories. Each category is also represented by a color; however, the name of the category and not the color should be used when referring to the category. Those in the immediate category are represented by red, delayed by yellow, minimal by green, expectant by gray, and dead by black.

Lifesaving Interventions. In SALT triage, four lifesaving interventions should be considered during the initial casualty assessment. These can be applied quickly with minimal resources, should not require a rescuer to stay with the injured person, and are likely to have a significant impact on reducing morbidity and mortality.

➤ *Control major hemorrhage*: This can be done with tourniquets or by having another person or device apply direct pressure.

➤ *Consider opening the airway:* This should be done only with simple positioning maneuvers such as a jaw thrust or head tilt/chin lift; alternatively, a basic airway adjunct can be inserted. If the injured person is a child who is not breathing, the rescuer can consider giving the child 2 rescue breaths.

➤ *Perform chest decompression:* If the person has an obvious pneumothorax, the rescuer if trained to do so can consider providing chest needle decompression.

➤ *Provide chemical antidotes:* If a chemical exposure to nerve agent is suspected, the rescuer may also consider providing autoinjector antidotes.

None of these interventions should be performed if they are outside the rescuer's scope of practice or if any needed equipment is not immediately available.

Triage Categories. In working with the five SALT triage categories, it is important to keep in mind that *expectant* does not mean dead. Casualties assigned to this category must be treated respectfully and should receive comfort care or resuscitation when resources are available. During a serious disaster, expectant casualties will not be treated until other less severely injured casualties are stabilized. For most health responders, assigning a person to this category will be difficult, but providing comfort care may assist both the patient and the caregiver.

Deceased persons should be triaged and tagged accordingly to prevent repeat triage, as resources are limited. Bodies should not be moved to ensure evidence preservation. The only exception to this important rule is a situation in which moving a corpse is necessary to rescue a living person. The fatally injured are the last to be evacuated from the scene. The local medical examiner or coroner is typically responsible for the identification, transport, and aftercare of the bodies.

As depicted in Figure 6-2, SALT mass casualty triage is designed for handling large numbers of casualties to save the most lives possible during a mass casualty event. As time, resources, and conditions allow, all casualties are assessed medically and triaged accordingly. SALT is, at best, an imperfect process implemented under austere conditions. It is also a dynamic process that is constantly influenced by changes in a person's condition, scene conditions, resource availability, and time (each of which can change for better or worse). During a mass casualty situation, triage personnel will have at their disposal only

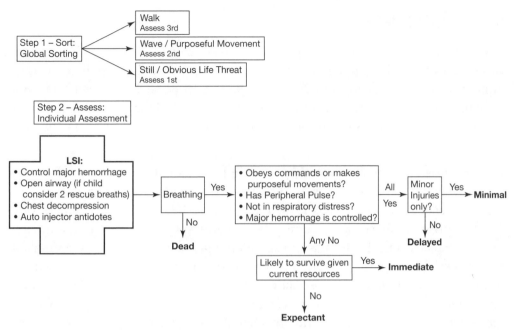

FIGURE 6-2 SALT Mass Casualty Triage

Source: Lerner EB, Schwartz RB, Coule PL, Weinstein ES, Cone DC, Hunt RC, et al. Mass casualty triage: an evaluation of the data and development of a proposed national guideline. Disaster Med and Public Health Prep. 2008;2(Suppl 1): S25–S34.

SALT Triage Categories

Category	Color Code	Description
Immediate	Red	Persons with critical injuries who have a good prognosis for survival given the resources available
Delayed	Yellow	Persons with significant injuries who are able to tolerate a delay in care without the risk of substantial morbidity
Minimal	Green	Persons whose injuries are minor enough that they can wait for treatment (eg, "walking wounded")
Expectant	Gray	Persons whose injuries are so severe that they have only a minimal chance of survival even if significant resources are expended; if resources become available, they should be treated as Immediate
Dead	Black	

their skills and judgment, and they will likely lack specialized equipment or tests. Their efforts will focus on the treatment of those persons who are most in need of care and most likely to benefit from it. The SALT Triage system and its application to various disaster situations is covered in much greater detail in the BDLS and ADLS courses.

6.9.3   Triage Tags

There is no single, unified system or tag design used in triage. Emergency responders should be familiar with the tag system used by their local EMS system, institution, or agency. Many products permit fairly detailed recording of a person's condition with color coding, bar codes for identification, vital signs, antidote administration, and even tagging of personal effects for later retrieval.

During disaster response, identification and documentation of casualties are vital. Even the most basic tag is the start of a casualty tracking system and medical record; therefore, it is critical to provide relevant information as time and resources allow. Triage tags may be in short supply or entirely unavailable in a particular event. In this case, responders may need to improvise with available materials and write directly on the person. For example, triage personnel might use markers or pens, lipstick, crime-scene tape or other tape, and examination gloves for recording pertinent clinical and historical information. No matter which method is used, the tag or label should be securely tied (or written) directly on the injured person, not to his or her clothing (which will be removed for decontamination, evaluation, or treatment). Further, tags should allow for the dynamic nature of triage and should allow for a triage category to be changed as the person's condition changes.

6.9.4   Population-Based Triage

To date, most disaster triage systems in the United States are based on mass casualty trauma situations and have limited application in large-scale disease outbreaks, in which triage decisions need to be based on infectiousness and duration of illness. Experience with the severe acute respiratory syndrome (SARS) outbreak in 2003 and other infectious disease outbreaks demonstrated the need for a population-based approach to triage that allows for prioritization of groups most in need of intervention to prevent or limit disease spread. A proposed triage model presumes that all populations share a common concern; that is, persons are either exposed and possibly infectious or unexposed and remain susceptible.[21] The goal of triage in an epidemic is to prevent secondary transmission through the implementation of nonmedical strategies (social distancing, shelter-in-place, isolation, quarantine, risk communication) and medical interventions (eg, immunization, medication, respiratory support). A population-based triage model, called *SEIRV*, has been proposed that is based on five triage categories:

➤ *Susceptible:* Persons who are not yet exposed but are susceptible

➤ *Exposed:* Persons who are susceptible and have been in contact with an infected person; they may be infected but are not yet contagious

➤ *Infectious:* Persons who are symptomatic and contagious

➤ *Removed:* Persons who no longer can transmit the disease to others because they have survived and developed immunity or died from the disease

➤ *Vaccinated* (or medicated): Persons who have received prophylactic medical intervention to protect them from infection

This system is discussed more in the BDLS and ADLS courses.

6.9.5   Casualty Assessment and Lifesaving Intervention

In any serious disaster or public health emergency, it is important to consider that the standard of care provided to all injured or ill persons may need to be altered. Communities and health facilities must plan and prepare for this reality by increasing citizen and staff awareness about this issue, as well as by creating an adequate legal framework to provide care during mass casualty events. In a serious disaster or public health emergency, the goal is to keep health systems functioning to deliver the highest level of care possible to save as many lives as possible. Recent guidance from the Agency for Health Research and Quality identifies four levels of medical standards that should be considered in all disaster plans to achieve this goal[22]:

➤ Normal medical standards

➤ Near-normal medical standards (eg, expanding the scope of practice for some response personnel, use of alternate care facilities, and atypical uses of certain medical equipment)

➤ Lifesaving care (eg, many casualties will only receive critical lifesaving intervention, nonessential services will be delayed or discontinued)

➤ Total systems/standards alteration (eg, severe rationing of care, some casualties receive no treatment)

In a disaster, delivery of care will depend on resources available at the scene. In a mass casualty event, health responders may have a difficult adjustment in making the shift from providing the best standard of care to individual patients sequentially, to providing the best possible standard of care to multiple patients simultaneously. During the initial response phase, treatment will often be limited to the most critical lifesaving and life-support interventions. Disaster treatment continues at the disaster scene until one of the following conditions is met:

➤ All patients have been transported; or

➤ Resources are exhausted.

After initial assessment, the most critically ill or injured persons with the greatest chance for survival will be given the highest priority for immediate care. Responders will determine those persons who are most in need of definitive medical care and prepare them for evacuation from the scene. Again, it is important to consider that the medical or trauma care provided at the scene may not be considered optimal, given the limited resources available.

Definitive medical care generally refers to care that will improve, rather than simply stabilize, the condition of a casualty (eg, surgical and critical care provided in a hospital). Requirements for definitive medical care will vary widely depending on the magnitude and epidemiology of the disaster. In some disasters, local hospitals may be destroyed or transportation to medical facilities might not be feasible. In such cases, hospital teams with mobile equipment might be organized and deployed to deliver medical care.

It is important to prevent all persons from leaving the disaster scene until they have been evaluated. Ideally, decontamination protocols should be implemented at the scene before emergency responders begin triage and treatment. Regardless of exposure to chemicals, radiation, or biologic agents, in the event of major or life-threatening traumatic injuries, casualties must be medically stabilized before any decontamination effort is made.

It is assumed that the student of this program has received the requisite training to provide lifesaving emergency care, and therefore this will not be repeated here. The specific and unique requirements of clinical care resulting from disasters is discussed in the BDLS course. It is important, however, that all responders learn that hemorrhage control from traumatic injuries is paramount. This may include applying tourniquets and pressure dressings to control hemorrhage.

First Aid Techniques to Learn and Practice

For those who are otherwise untrained, CPR and first aid courses offered by the American Red Cross, the American Heart Association, and other community organizations can prove valuable to rendering assistance during an emergency. During a disaster many victims can result that overwhelm the health system and therefore bystanders and even other victims may be called upon to provide assistance and first aid care. Of these controlling bleeding is paramount. Serious bleeding from injuries can be life threatening if not controlled. Below is a list of interventions to control bleeding:

➤ Apply direct pressure to the wound

➤ Elevate the wounded part above the level of the heart

➤ Apply a pressure dressing with compression wrap (ace-wrap or similar)

➤ When serious bleeding from an arm or leg can not be controlled with the measures above a tourniquet can be applied to control bleeding by those who are trained.

Nonmedical personnel should all be trained in first aid techniques to render assistance during a disaster. Contact the American Red Cross or other organizations concerning formal first aid training.

6.9.6   Public Health Assessment and Intervention

In a disaster, affected individuals and communities must have their basic physiologic and psychological needs met in a timely manner. Public health authorities will perform a rapid needs assessment to determine the magnitude of the event, the impact on essential services (including potable water supply, sanitation capacity, food supply, shelter, and electricity), and local health response capacities. This includes establishing priorities, standards, and monitoring systems for water, food, sanitation and solid waste removal, shelter, animal and vector control, and communicable disease control. Public health professionals will work with emergency response agencies to ensure that affected populations are aware of health and safety risks and how to either avoid them or prepare to deal with them. Throughout the event, public health personnel will focus on the bigger picture, that is, getting the community back to health. The role of the public health system in responding to disasters and public health emergencies is discussed in greater detail in the BDLS and ADLS courses.

The initial response to large-scale infectious disease outbreaks (such as an influenza pandemic) will focus on containing the spread of the disease, if feasible, through individual- and population-based measures that can help slow transmission. Aggressive and sustained public health surveillance will be a cornerstone public health function. Today, extensive international and domestic travel and the interdependence between countries, states, and communities make it unlikely that strict movement restrictions could be imposed effectively to limit disease spread. Containment strategies aimed at controlling and slowing the spread of the disease might include measures that affect individuals (eg, hand hygiene, cough etiquette, isolation, and monitoring of contacts) as well as measures that affect groups or entire communities (eg, cancellation of public gatherings, closing of schools and businesses). Evacuations will most likely have no meaningful effect on the spread of disease and probably will be counterproductive (ie, they will merely move a group of people likely to require services and health care to another site that is already overburdened or soon to be overburdened). The use of vaccines and antimicrobial medications will also be an important consideration.

6.9.7   Special Health Considerations

No two disasters are identical. Many different situations can arise that call for special considerations, perhaps a slight variance from the norm, or an adjustment to preparedness plans. The United States is a multicultural and multilingual society, and it is very possible that people from various cultural and religious backgrounds may require assistance from rescuers and responders who are not familiar with their cultural and religious customs. Disaster responders also may be confronted with familial and language issues that impede access to medication histories, delivery of health records, and administration of vaccinations. Attention to empathy, compassion, and decency can help overcome most of these concerns.

Issues regarding the triage and treatment of special-needs populations such as children, pregnant women, frail elderly, and disabled persons should be addressed well in advance of a disaster. It is important to include these groups as well as cultural competency issues in predisaster planning. Triage categories should be referred to by their name (immediate, delayed, minimal, expectant, dead) as opposed to the color representing the category, as this could be confused as referring to a race or ethnic group. A reasonably accurate disaster plan can help forecast the needs of particular populations and community groups during different disaster scenarios. The young and old alike have unique needs when it comes to medical attention and service in a disaster. Children are not small adults, and consideration should be given to medication dosages and equipment sizing, as well as for water temperature and methods of decontamination should the need arise.

6.10   EVACUATION

Evacuation may be defined as the timely and orderly removal of injured and uninjured people from the disaster scene and affected region. These people could include:

➤ Injured

➤ Uninjured with no means of transport

➤ Rescue personnel

➤ Families of casualties

➤ Patients in hospitals

➤ Community at large

Planning and preparing for individual and community evacuation needs; understanding the target population, their concerns and nuances; and knowing where they can be safely relocated to during a disaster, all play an important role in community disaster preparedness. Evacuations should be a commonly exercised component of all disaster plans. The number of people to be evacuated, the modes of transportation, and the rapidity with which the evacuation occurs vary with the situation at hand. Evacuation plans must account for complex scenarios, such as the evacuation of schools, high-rises, hospitals, and chronic care facilities, (eg, nursing homes and rehabilitation facilities). Evacuation of schools requires not only close supervision and direction of a large number of young children, but also a coordinated effort to contact parents and arrange for reunification with parents and pickup if necessary. High-rise structure evacuations create significant logistical challenges for rescue workers. The inability to use elevators and the limited number of stairwells are just two of the many difficulties encountered in these situations. Evacuation plans should also include preparations to prevent panicked loved ones who arrive on scene from interfering with rescue efforts or becoming potential casualties.

Schools and businesses should have evacuation plans that include processes and procedures to document individuals who leave the premises and move to a safer location. Plans should also be developed, practiced, and implemented for casualties evacuated from the disaster scene. All persons transported to area hospitals or alternate care facilities should be identified at the scene, so they can be accounted for and tracked. Records should indicate all area facilities that receive casualties. Mechanisms must be in place to help relatives, neighbors, and emergency management personnel identify persons who may still be in danger and require assistance. This includes mechanisms to help reunite families and loved ones after an event, as well as assist efforts to identify missing persons.

Evacuation planning includes making community members aware of their personal need for preparedness. Community members should be encouraged to participate in disaster preparedness plans and practice drills to inform them about local evacuation procedures. As discussed in Chapter 2 of this manual, individuals and families should be encouraged to plan ahead and assemble a disaster readiness kit.

6.10.1   Pre-event Evacuation

The goal of pre-event evacuation is to prevent injury. When community evacuations are necessary, local government officials can provide warning methods for evacuation through the local media (radio and television reports), sirens, telephone calls, and direct contact and communication. Any instructions given should be followed closely. If instructed to evacuate immediately due to impending danger, individuals should gather household essentials and leave the premises.

Determinations need to be made about the safety of evacuation routes to facilitate the movements desired. Questions that need to be addressed include:

➤ Is evacuation the best course, or should shelter-in-place be considered?

➤ Where will populations be evacuated to?

➤ How will they get there?

➤ Who will manage and communicate updates to them while they are temporarily housed?

➤ What about animals? (Many people simply will not leave without the family pet.)

In pre-event evacuation, the majority of individuals will not need medical or assisted transport and will evacuate or avail themselves of emergency management directed mass transportation resources. A percentage of the affected population will include persons with disabilities, the elderly, and occupants of hospitals and chronic care and rehabilitation facilities. These individuals will need a combination of assisted and medical evacuation. Consideration also must be given to pre-event evacuation of pets and livestock.

Resourceful and creative evacuation options are the key to transportation preparedness. If a disaster can be monitored or can be predicted, then elected leaders can order and execute an evacuation before the event occurs, usually on the advice of emergency managers. It can take days to evacuate a large city and therefore the timeline before impact of the event must be considered. This will allow individuals to escape unharmed in a timely fashion and allow a more orderly evacuation as routes and resources may not yet be limited by the event. Examples include a forest fire encroaching on a nearby neighborhood several miles away or a distant hurricane. Unfortunately, in many other disaster situations such as earthquakes, chemical release, bombings, and nuclear explosions, there is no warning and the disaster may be completely unexpected.

6.10.2 Postevent Evacuation

The expeditious evacuation of injured and uninjured individuals to a safer environment should receive top priority in any disaster situation. Timely, orderly, and efficient evacuation can involve substantial organizational and logistical challenges, especially because many disasters occur without prior warning. In postevent evacuation, some of the individuals who are uninjured may be able to self-evacuate under direction from incident command, but many will need either assisted evacuation or medical evacuation. Initial evacuation is a coordinated effort among multiple local agencies, particularly police, fire, and EMS, under the direction of the incident commander. In the terrorist attacks of September 11, 2001, most survivors required evacuation within the first minutes or hours after the event.[23] A second wave of survivors, composed largely of rescue personnel, followed. Few survivors were rescued or required evacuation more than 24 hours after the event.

Evacuation does not require EMS ambulance transport for all injured persons. The disposition options for injured persons include treatment and release from the scene, transportation to area hospitals, and transport to secondary hospitals. A top priority is to avoid overwhelming the closest hospitals. Equitable and rational distribution of casualties among available regional facilities reduces the burden on each hospital to a manageable level, potentially even to nondisaster levels. Transport officials should have a good working knowledge of regional hospital and transport capabilities to distribute casualties throughout the region. People with burns, pediatric casualties, those with multisystem trauma, and certain injuries requiring hyperbaric therapy should be sent to the appropriate specialty hospital. Stable persons with minor injuries should be distributed evenly and equitably among medical centers in the region. Ideally, balanced casualty distribution would be achieved via a centrally controlled EMS system working with the incident command.

Transport in a devastated urban area will be very difficult because of damaged infrastructure. Evacuation routes recommended by emergency personnel should be followed, as usual shortcuts may be blocked because of hazardous conditions. Critical egress routes and backup alternate routes should be identified in advance, but they also may be unavailable after an event. Public transportation vehicles, school buses, airport car rental shuttle buses, police cars, and taxis can be used to evacuate people from the scene. Air evacuation is a limited resource and may not be available during severe weather or when the civil authorities close airspace as they did during September 11, 2001.

Special provisions need to be made to move disabled, elderly, and dispossessed (eg, homeless) persons, children, and institutional populations such as those in schools, hospitals, and prisons. Hospital evacuations are often facilitated by predetermined mutual aid agreements with other community medical facilities. These agreements may increase capacity for personnel, equipment, or space for evacuated patients. Hospital evacuation challenges are compounded when the structure is a high-rise. The evacuation of a "stable" ventilator patient from an intensive care unit, down several flights of stairs, using manual/portable means to provide respiratory support, while continuing critical intravenous medications is very challenging. The potential for increased morbidity, mortality, and liability in these situations is significant.

Specific information targeted to special needs groups, such as children, the elderly, the disabled, and pet owners, is available.[24,25] Government agencies, the American Red Cross, the Salvation Army, and other disaster relief organizations may be able to provide temporary shelter and emergency supplies. It is also important to consider how the community will respond to increased demand for medical supplies. The community must plan for and expect an increase in lost medications, worsened medical conditions, and a general increase in the demand for medications.

6.11 RECOVERY

After a disaster, the immediate impact of physical injury and the loss to life, personal property, and the community can be overwhelming. The overall goal of recovery is to restore the community to a "normal" level of functioning and minimize the impact of the event. Effective preparation can significantly reduce the stressors associated with any catastrophic situation and may facilitate the recovery process. In many disaster situations, the problem is not the lack of resources but the lack of coordination between responding agencies. A well-exercised disaster preparedness plan can help mitigate some of these problems and lead to improved recovery.

Recovery is the longest phase of any disaster and begins when the event occurs. The recovery phase requires a long-term commitment to the affected communities. In terms of physical, economic, and community recovery, this phase may take months or years. The physical and psychological imprint from a disaster can last a lifetime for some affected individuals. Government agencies, businesses, and various organizations (eg, American Red Cross, the Salvation Army) work together to provide community support during this period.

Recovery is a process that cannot be rushed. Recovery can mean different things to different people: to families it may mean reestablishment in their home; to a businessperson it means getting the store open again and everyone their jobs back. To the community at large, it may mean a feeling of closure, a time to heal from the event, and a time to rebuild. There may be legal proceedings that need to take place, often months or years after the event, that will delay ultimate closure and recovery. Community members can and should be involved in the recovery process. Collectively, they can take steps to understand what has happened and why, and can think about what needs to be done to prevent or mitigate repeat occurrences.

As described in Chapters 2 and 3 of this manual, preparedness is critical for the expeditious recovery of damaged or disrupted homes, businesses, and communities. Pre-event mitigation, with attention to construction practices, building location, and engineering principles, should be an important component of business and community disaster planning. Controls and backup systems should be in place to help mitigate problems that arise during a disaster (eg, power loss). Ideally, businesses and residences should be built in low-risk areas (ie, away from flood zones) and designed to meet building codes applicable to local hazards (eg, earthquakes, wind).

6.11.1   The Immediate Recovery Period

In the immediate aftermath of a disaster, preservation of life is the primary goal. Depending on the type of disaster, local rescue efforts and medical facilities may be overwhelmed or incapacitated. The recovery phase of a disaster requires a coordinated effort by multiple agencies such as local government officials, police, fire service, EMS, and area hospitals. Reestablishing local health care delivery is a priority in the initial recovery period.

Depending on the disaster, there could be a significant number of newly homeless or severely resource-impaired families. Providing adequate shelter and facility access to all affected populations is important. Food, water, shelter, and clothing are basic needs of everyone in the community. Other major problems that should be anticipated immediately after a disaster include disruption in telecommunication systems (ie, both land-based and cellular), utilities, and computer systems. Not only do coordinated backup capabilities need to be considered, but individuals responding to a disaster need to be educated on how to use these systems.

The news media is a valuable resource for disseminating vital information and may assist recovery efforts. Television and radio broadcasts can be used to help solicit additional help from volunteers and businesses, as well as to inform the public about how to get in touch with loved ones and inform onlookers about dangerous areas to avoid. A preestablished agreement with the local media is helpful, and a single point for information release should be established.

6.11.2 Recovery Beyond the Immediate Period

Between 3 and 7 days after a disaster, management of the initial wave of casualties will be nearly complete. Reestablishment of local health care resources and other critical infrastructure will become the primary focus. Uninjured people who have had delays in accessing the local health system will increasingly seek and demand access. People with chronic illnesses and special needs patients who have depleted or lost their medications, experienced interrupted home health care service, exhausted special supplies such as oxygen or insulin, or have a multitude of other needs will seek medical care.

This increased patient volume coupled with a damaged or compromised infrastructure can be difficult for the local health community to manage. During this time, Disaster Medical Assistance Team (DMAT) assistance is vital. DMAT teams are experts in decompressing an overburdened local health system. In addition to caring for immediate treatment of casualties, DMAT teams have the capacity to provide primary care and other basic priority services. Disaster Mortuary Operational Response Teams (DMORTs) can be a valuable resource for any disasters involving mass fatalities.

If the event is the result of a criminal act, law enforcement officials will pursue the apprehension and successful prosecution of the perpetrator(s). Forensic investigation should proceed in parallel with other recovery functions. Other response agencies (eg, public health, mental health) should respect and assist law enforcement investigations as needed. Such assistance may include preservation of the chain of custody or other actions to protect evidence for subsequent prosecution. Law enforcement activities may directly affect public health; for example, apprehension of the perpetrator may halt the ongoing release of a biologic agent into the environment. Successful law enforcement also can contribute to the mental well-being of the affected population. Apprehension of the perpetrator(s) can impart feelings that justice is being served and provide a positive psychological impact for affected individuals, their families, and the community at large.

For federally declared disasters, Disaster Recovery Centers established by FEMA are available to assist individuals and communities in their struggle to rebuild their lives and return to a normal level of functioning.[26] Individuals can meet face-to-face with representatives from federal, state, local, and volunteer agencies that can assist them in obtaining resources to help with the rebuilding effort. Businesses may apply to the Small Business Administration for possible assistance in declared disaster areas.[27]

DisasterAssistance.gov

In the wake of Hurricane Katrina in 2005, hundreds of thousands of people needed emergency assistance, such as housing, food, and clothing. An executive order was issued in response to that disaster requiring the federal government to simplify the process of identifying and applying for assistance.

In response to the executive order, DisasterAssistance.gov was created as a secure Web portal to consolidate disaster assistance information in one location. Affected persons who need assistance after a presidentially declared disaster can go to this Web site to register online. Informational resources are also available to help citizens learn about various disaster assistance programs and services. Currently, 17 US government agencies, which sponsor almost 60 forms of assistance, contribute to the portal. DisasterAssistance.gov facilitates the application process by feeding common data to multiple online applications in a secure environment. This includes applications for FEMA assistance and referral to the Small Business Administration for loans through online applications.

For more information, refer to http://www.disasterassistance.gov.

Local public health agencies play a vital role in the recovery period. Public health personnel will oversee long-term surveillance of affected populations to identify physiologic and psychological effects from the event, ensure continuity of health operations, and ensure implementation of changes generated from a systematic evaluation of health system response efforts. Accurate assessment of community health needs must be based on valid data. Speculation and assumptions can be financially costly and damaging to the recovery efforts. Effective public health surveillance mechanisms must be implemented and sustained.

6.11.3   Mental Health Impact of Disasters

The psychological impact of any disaster is an important consideration during the recovery phase. A critical first step in reducing the mental health impact of a disaster is an effective risk communication plan. A spokesperson should be identified who is credible and trusted and who can provide accurate and frequent assessments of what is and what is not known. To reduce population fear and anxiety, rumors should be anticipated and debunked as quickly as possible.

Providing for the mental health needs of affected individuals, their families, and emergency response workers is an essential function of crisis management. Feelings of anxiety, sadness, grief, and anger are normal reactions to any disaster event. If the event is a result of an intentional or terrorist act, these normal reactions can be exacerbated. Appropriate counseling may reduce suicide risks, work absenteeism, and chronic disease exacerbations attributed to stress and other behavioral and emotional reactions to the event. Early intervention will minimize long-term negative psychological outcomes. For rescue workers and health providers, a debriefing about the incident should take place in the immediate period after any disaster. Workers should be assessed for behaviors that may warrant further evaluation and assistance from a qualified mental health professional.

Restoration of mental health after a disaster may be a prolonged process. The effect on mental health may extend well beyond those who directly experienced the disaster, perhaps significantly involving those who witnessed events via television or other media. Acute stress disorder may be common among both victims and responders. With appropriate treatment, including emphasis on the normal recovery process (talking to others, getting rest and respite, and returning to normal routines), recovery may be facilitated.

6.11.4 Special Population Considerations

During recovery, special consideration needs to be given to special populations such as non–English-speaking persons, children, the elderly, those who have specific medical needs, and those with limited means such as the homeless or those living in poverty.

➤ Various groups in the United States have belief systems and customs specific to their religion or culture. These customs and beliefs, such as the disposition of remains from a mass fatality incident, may conflict with the recovery process. Inclusion of all relevant cultures and customs should be incorporated into the all-hazards disaster planning process, which will provide for a collaborative plan that addresses specific populations and their needs.

➤ The elderly often have multiple health issues that require skilled health personnel and specialized medical equipment and supplies. Steps need to be taken to ensure continuity of health care and medications for the elderly during the recovery period. In addition, family members and other caregivers must be aware of indicators that the elderly are not handling the stress of the situation appropriately.

➤ Many important differences distinguish children from adults, which is the origin of the often-used phrase, "children are not small adults." Children have many unique anatomic, physiologic, immunologic, developmental, and psychological considerations that potentially affect their vulnerability to injury and response in a disaster. It is important to account for these vulnerabilities before an event in disaster planning, as well as after an event in triage, diagnosis, management, and recovery.

➤ Individuals of lower socioeconomic status present additional challenges. Many rely on governmental assistance and lack the resources to recover from a disaster. Included in this category are the homeless or near-homeless that may not have access to the normal outlets of communication such as radio, Internet, or television. Disaster planning needs to include a method to reach this population.

➤ Non–English-speaking populations pose a challenge in disaster recovery. These populations must be identified and communicated with, and they must be provided with the necessary instructions on available resources.

➤ Consideration must be given to those with special medical needs who may require additional assistance and who may be displaced. A greater number of medical and human resources are required to assist people with special health needs, such as additional equipment and supplies, as well as properly trained providers and volunteers to assist with everyday tasks such as personal care, hygiene, ambulation, and rehabilitation.

6.11.5   Business and Industry Considerations

Economic impacts, coupled with damage to building and transportation infrastructure, can be difficult for the local businesses to manage. Beyond meeting the needs of the employees they serve, senior and executive staff must think about business continuity to keep the organization running during and after the event. Again, a well-written and well-practiced disaster plan is essential to prepare for, respond to, and recover from disasters and other serious emergencies.

An additional need in the disaster recovery process is recovery assistance for businesses in the affected community. It is generally acknowledged that approximately 50% of businesses will not return after a disaster. This results in a cascading financial impact due to loss of employment and insurance coverage for workers, loss of tax revenue for communities, financial instability, and the resulting loss of commerce for other area businesses. The federal government provides assistance through FEMA grants for federally declared disasters. In addition, the Small Business Administration assists businesses, homeowners, and renters with reduced-rate and extended-term loans to assist reentry of businesses after a disaster. Small Business Development Centers serve as a regional resource by bringing together the private sector, the educational sector, and the government to assist in the recovery process.

6.11.6   Postincident Analysis and Reporting

Thorough postevent analysis and issuance of an after-action report are imperative to determine the overall successes and shortfalls of the disaster management system. By revisiting the event, beginning with the disaster plan, and studying what went right and where improvement opportunities exist, emergency planners and managers can be better prepared for future events. Were the assumptions in the disaster plan accurate? Did the ICS work as exercised? The questions are many, but the opportunity they present for learning about the overall response to improve future responses is worth the effort. The community needs to be brought back not only to where it was before the event but, by applying lessons learned, to a better state. When recovery is built into the planning process, thought about during mitigation, and considered during the response, this ultimate goal is attainable.

NIMS includes resources for post-incident analysis, critique, and lessons learned. Having a consistent approach for all phases of emergency and disaster management makes collaborative learning and information-sharing among multiple agencies and organizations a real possibility and a staple in strengthening national disaster preparedness.

6.12 SUMMARY

When one considers the catastrophic possibilities that a disaster may potentially present, the limited personnel and resources that will likely be on hand in the initial response phase, the limited experience many people will ever have facing a disaster situation, and the pressure that all of these factors will collectively represent, then one can begin to comprehend the value of the DISASTER Paradigm. It is more than just another acronym or mnemonic. The DISASTER Paradigm provides a practical framework that can be applied and utilized in all phases of disaster management, but particularly during the response phase when time is critical and resources are limited.

Detection requires awareness of the environment, recognition of unusual circumstances, and, in some cases, a high index of suspicion. For natural disasters, nuclear detonations, and explosive events, prediction can be difficult or impossible, but detection after the event is very straightforward. For chemical emergencies, detection hinges on environmental clues and on familiarity with the characteristic presentations (toxidromes) of the major chemical classes. For biologic agents, environmental clues, patient symptoms, disease syndromes, and careful surveillance are critical. For radiologic disasters, early detection may be difficult, especially for a covert release.

Incident management can be facilitated through the incorporation of NIMS and ICS principles for managing time, personnel, and resources in any size emergency or disaster. The importance of implementing a command structure from the very outset of an event cannot be overemphasized.

Safety and security in a disaster are dynamic, ever changing as the situation unfolds. Vigilance is paramount.

Assessment of real and potential hazards related to an evolving scene must be done continually.

Support from multiple agencies and organizations is critical. Understanding how local, state, and federal emergency plans coordinate, align, and work in conjunction with one another can help a great deal in understanding what resources can be expected from whom, and over what time frame.

Triage and treatment of casualties in a disaster is about identifying critically injured and salvageable casualties and rendering lifesaving interventions.

Evacuation involves population movement before or after disaster strikes. Thoughtful planning for evacuation can attenuate risk before and after a disaster.

Recovery is a long-term process. It is complete when the community and its members have returned to normal, pre-event functioning. This may take many years and may never be fully realized. Psychosocial and mental health challenges following a disaster contribute to a need for crisis management for individuals, families, and response personnel. Extensive and appropriate local, regional, federal, and nongovernmental resources contribute to the recovery process.

Throughout the NDLS courses and related training programs, it is important to continuously reinforce the message that, regardless of the disaster cause, first responders and health workers must protect their personal health and safety at all times to avoid becoming casualties themselves.

6.13 SELF-LEARNING SCENARIOS

After completing the CDLS course and each of the chapters in this manual, take time to work through the 4 scenarios presented in Appendix A. The scenarios are designed for the application and reinforcement of "core" concepts and principles in disaster life support.

REFERENCES

1. Federal Communications Commission. Emergency alert system. http://www.fcc.gov/pshs/services/eas/. Accessed September 21, 2009.

2. National Weather Service. NOAA Weather Radio All Hazards. http://www.weather.gov/nwr/. Accessed September 21, 2009.

3. Centers for Disease Control and Prevention. Recognition of illness associated with the intentional release of a biologic agent. *MMWR Morb Mortal Wkly Rep.* 2001;50:893–897. http://www.cdc.gov/mmwr/preview/mmwrhtml/mm5041a2.htm. Accessed September 21, 2009.

4. Weinstein RS, Alibek K, eds. *Biological and Chemical Terrorism: A Guide for Healthcare Workers and First Responders*. New York, NY: Thieme Medical Publishers Inc; 2003:11.

5. Centers for Disease Control and Prevention. Recognition of illness associated with exposure to chemical agents—United States, 2003. *MMWR Morb Mortal Wkly Rep*. 2003;52:938–940. http://www.cdc.gov/mmwr/preview/mmwrhtml/mm5239a3.htm. Accessed September 21, 2009.

6. Federal Emergency Management Agency. NIMS Resource Center. http://www.fema.gov/emergency/nims/. Accessed September 21, 2009.

7. FIRESCOPE. http://firescope.org/. Accessed September 21, 2009.

8. California Emergency Medical Services Authority. Disaster Medical Services Division—Hospital Incident Command System (HICS). http://www.emsa.ca.gov/hics/. Accessed September 21, 2009.

9. Occupational Safety and Health Administration. Safety and health topics: personal protective equipment. http://www.osha.gov/SLTC/personalprotectiveequipment/. Accessed September 21, 2009.

10. Assistant Secretary for Preparedness and Response, US Department of Health and Human Services. National Disaster Medical System. http://www.hhs.gov/aspr/opeo/ndms/index.html. Accessed September 21, 2009.

11. Centers for Disease Control and Prevention. Strategic National Stockpile. http://www.bt.cdc.gov/stockpile/. Accessed September 21, 2009.

12. Phillips SJ, Knebel A, Johnson K, eds. *Mass Medical Care With Scarce Resources: The Essentials*. AHRQ publication 09-0016. Rockville, MD: Agency for Healthcare Research and Quality; 2009. http://www.ahrq.gov/prep/mmcessentials/mccessent.pdf. Accessed September 21, 2009.

13. National Center for Injury Prevention and Control. *In a Moment's Notice: Surge Capacity for Terrorist Bombings*. Atlanta, GA: Centers for Disease Control and Prevention; 2007. http://www.bt.cdc.gov/masscasualties/pdf/surgecapacity.pdf. Accessed September 21, 2009.

14. US Department of Health and Human Services. Disasters and emergencies, Appendix D: Glossary. http://www.hhs.gov/disasters/discussion/planners/mscc/appendix/d.html. Accessed December 11, 2009.

15. American Academy of Pediatrics; Foltin GL, Schonfeld DJ, Shannon MW, eds. *Terrorism and Disaster Preparedness: A Resource for Pediatricians*. AHRQ publication 06(07)-0056. Rockville, MD: Agency for Healthcare Research and Quality; October 2006. http://www.ahrq.gov/RESEARCH/PEDPREP/pedresource.pdf. Accessed September 21, 2009.

16. Lerner EB, Schwartz RB, Coule PL, et al. Mass casualty triage: an evaluation of the data and development of a proposed national guideline. *Disaster Med Public Health Prep*. 2008;2(suppl 1):S25–S34.

17. Cone D, MacMillan D. Mass casualty triage systems: a hint of science. *Acad Emerg Med*. 2005;12:739–741.

18. Newport Beach Fire Department (Newport Beach, California). START triage. http://www.start-triage.com/. Accessed September 21, 2009.

19. Romig LE. The JumpSTART Pediatric MCI Triage Tool. http://www.jumpstarttriage.com/. Accessed September 21, 2009.

20. SALT mass casualty triage: concept endorsed by the American College of Emergency Physicians, American College of Surgeons Committee on Trauma, American Trauma Society, National Association of EMS Physicians, National Disaster Life Support Education Consortium, and State and Territorial Injury Prevention Directors Association. *Disaster Med Public Health Prep*. 2008;2:245–246.

21. Burkle FM. Mass casualty management of a large scale bioterrorist event: an epidemiological approach that shapes triage decisions. *Emerg Med Clin North Am*. 2002;20:409–436.

22. Agency for Healthcare Research and Quality. *Altered Standards of Care in Mass Casualty Events: Bioterrorism and Other Public Health Emergencies*. Publication 05-0043. Rockville, MD: AHRQ; 2005. http://www.ahrq.gov/research/altstand/. Accessed September 21, 2009.

23. Rapid assessment of injuries among survivors of the terrorist attack on the World Trade Center—New York City, September 2001. *MMWR Morb Mortal Wkly Rep*. 2002;51:1–5. http://www.cdc.gov/mmwr/preview/mmwrhtml/mm5101a1.htm. Accessed September 21, 2009.

24. American Red Cross. http://www.redcross.org/. Accessed September 21, 2009.

25. US Department of Homeland Security. Ready. http://www.ready.gov/. Accessed September 21, 2009.

26. Federal Emergency Management Agency. About DRCs. http://www.fema.gov/assistance/opendrcs.shtm. Accessed September 21, 2009.

27. US Small Business Administration. http://www.sba.gov/. Accessed September 21, 2009.

GLOSSARY

All-hazards preparedness: Planning that considers all potential hazards to a community and taking steps to mitigate, practice, and respond to any potential hazard that may affect the community

Alternative care sites: Facilities that can be used in a disaster to care for "overflow" patients transferred from large hospitals and trauma centers to make room in these facilities for more acutely injured people. Such sites may include rehabilitation hospitals, nursing homes, and community health centers

Bioterrorism: Use of a living organism such as a virus or bacteria (or its products) against a civilian population to enact terrorism

Capacity assessment: Identifying available resources that can be used to reduce risk, enhance survival, and help affected individuals and populations cope with severe trauma

Chemical terrorism: Use of chemical agents (eg, sarin, mustard, phosgene), or the release of industrial chemicals (eg, chlorine, ammonia), to enact terrorism

Competencies: Abilities and skills of both public and private sector agents of public health legal preparedness in accessing and understanding the relevant laws and applying them to given health issues

Conflict-based disaster: An intentional, human-caused disaster event such as those related to war or terrorism

Containment: Defining and containing an outbreak in specific geographic regions

Coordination: Law-based action across multiple jurisdictions and within the constitutional and political framework

DISASTER Paradigm™: A mnemonic that organizes the providers' response and planning of a disaster: D, detect; I, incident management; S, security and safety;

A, assess hazards; S, support; T, triage and treatment; E, evacuation; R, recovery

Disaster supply kit: A collection of basic items that family members may need in a disaster, including adequate food, water, and other supplies to last for at least 3 days, and, if possible, for up to 2 weeks

Disaster: A serious disruption of the functioning of society, causing widespread human, material, or environmental losses that exceed the ability of affected society to cope by using only its own resources (World Association of Disaster and Emergency Medicine); an occurrence of a natural catastrophe, technological accident, or human-caused event that has resulted in severe property damage, deaths, and/or multiple injuries (FEMA); an event and its consequences that results in a serious disruption of the functioning of a community and causing widespread human, material, economic, or environmental losses that exceed the capacity of the affected area to respond without external assistance to save lives, preserve property, and maintain the stability and integrity of the affected area (NDLS Education Consortium)

Dual-use capacity: The ability of a system to provide ongoing trauma care at all levels as well as being ready to ramp up to meet disaster conditions, thereby helping to organize the disaster response

Emergency management: Coordination and integration of all activities necessary to build, sustain, and improve the capability to prepare for, protect against, respond to, recover from, or mitigate against threatened or actual natural disasters, acts of terrorism, or other human-caused disasters

Emergency operations center (EOC): Physical location where the leaders of a region or organization come together during an emergency or disaster to analyze response and recovery options, coordinate actions, and allocate resources

Essential public health services: Clean water, sanitation, food, health services, shelter, fuel, disease surveillance capability

Excess mortality and morbidity: Deaths and illnesses, indirectly resulting from a disaster, that would have been preventable had the need for public health measures been predicted or managed

External disaster: Anything that indirectly affects an institution's infrastructure

Hazard assessment: Analyzing various hazards for a particular geographic area and the magnitude of impact given local resources, allowing for prioritization of response and mitigation options

Hazard vulnerability assessment: Identifying particular infrastructures and populations at increased risk for damage or harm, which may affect local operations

Hazard: Anything that has the potential to do harm to property, the environment, people, or animals

Health disaster: a precipitous or gradual decline in the overall health status of a community for which the community is unable to cope without outside assistance

ICE: Acronym for "in case of emergency," used to designate a telephone number stored in an individual's cellular telephone for use by emergency responders if the individual is ill or injured

ID-MED: Mnemonic for the five categories of triage under the SALT method: immediate, delayed, minimal, expectant, and dead

Incident management: The way in which incidents are managed across all Homeland Security activities, including prevention, protection, response, mitigation, and recovery

Internal disaster: Condition that affects a facility directly (such a building fire); may be an extension of an external disaster

Isolation: Placement of persons known to have a communicable disease in a separate area where they will not expose others

Laws or legal authorities: Statutes, ordinances, judicial rulings, policies, executive orders, administrative rules and regulations, memoranda of understanding, and mutual aid agreements

Mitigation planning: Planning aimed at lessening the severity and impact of a potential emergency

National Incident Management System (NIMS): A comprehensive, national approach to incident management that is applicable at all jurisdictional levels and across functional disciplines

Natural disaster: Term used for a naturally occurring event or hazard that results in a disaster

Nuclear terrorism: Intentional detonation of nuclear weapons

Pandemic: A new infectious disease that emerges to which the population has little or no immunity

Population-based care: Decision making that considers the well-being of entire communities and populations

PRE-DISASTER Paradigm™: Steps to take before a disaster occurs: P, planning and practice; R, resilience; E, education

Preparedness planning: Development of resources and organizational capacity to prevent or manage the effects of a disaster on the basis of local risk assessments

Principle of autonomy: Right to self-determination, the need to justify infringements on individual rights, and the need to balance individuals' freedoms should they compete and/or conflict

Principle of beneficence: Duty to promote individual and public welfare through the maximizing of benefits and minimizing of harms

Principle of justice: Equitable distribution of benefits and risks

Principle of nonmaleficence: Active avoidance of harming patients and communities

Public health: A complex network of people, systems, and organizations that work together to ensure the conditions necessary to live healthy lives

Push packages: Caches of pharmaceuticals, antidotes, and medical supplies designed to provide rapid delivery of a broad spectrum of assets for an ill-defined threat in the early hours of an event

Quarantine: Placement of persons exposed to a contagious disease, but currently asymptomatic, in a separate area where they will not expose others and can be monitored for the development of the disease

Radiological terrorism: Use of radioactive materials to enact terrorism; usually refers to an intentional "dirty" bomb release, which is an explosive laced with a radioactive material such as cesium 137

Recovery planning: Planning for continuity of operations, restoration of essential services and infrastructure, and resumption of normal social and economic activities with minimal delay after a disaster

Response planning: Planning how local agencies and organizations will be engaged and mobilized when a disaster occurs

Risk perception: Understanding how different people perceive and measure risk

Risk: The probability of a potential hazard actually occurring

SALT: Proposed national standard for mass casualty triage; stands for *s*ort, *a*ssess, *l*ifesaving interventions, and *t*reatment and/or transport

SEIRV: Population-based triage method for infectious illness; stands for *s*usceptible, *e*xposed, *i*nfectious, *r*emoved, and *v*accinated

Social distancing: A disease prevention strategy in which a community imposes limitations on social (face-to-face) interactions to reduce exposure to and transmission of a virus

Special needs population, vulnerable population: Terms used interchangeably to characterize groups whose needs are not fully addressed by traditional service providers

Surge capacity: The ability of a health care system to rapidly expand beyond normal services to meet the increased demand for care of patients, which may include physical space or hospital beds, qualified personnel, medical care, and public health services

Technological disaster: An event resulting from a human systems failure, such as poorly designed buildings or flawed equipment, and human errors due to inadequate training, worker distraction, or fatigue

Terrorism: Use of chemical, biological, radiological, nuclear, and explosive agents to coerce, intimidate, or cause panic

Time-limited disaster: A disaster less than 72 hours in duration. Also called mass casualty incident (MCI; local, five or more patients) or mass casualty event (MCE; regional, 20 or more patients)

Toxidrome: A typical, specific set of signs and symptoms caused by a given chemical class

Triage: Prioritization of care for patients based on the severity of their illness or injury, their ability to survive, and the resources available

Appendices

CDLS® Self-Learning Scenarios

Four applied learning scenarios have been developed to supplement and reinforce content presented in the CDLS course and course manual. These include a:

➤ Major hurricane

➤ Hazardous materials release

➤ Influenza pandemic

➤ Terrorist bombing

The scenarios include content relevant to multiple response professions and are designed to stimulate thinking among all persons who may find themselves working together in an emergency situation. The purpose of these scenarios is to provide course participants with the opportunity to demonstrate that they retained and can apply knowledge by allowing them to problem-solve within the constraints of CDLS course material. Before looking at the self-learning scenarios, participants should complete the CDLS course and read the course manual.

MAJOR HURRICANE

Learning Objective.   After completing this scenario, you will be able to apply the principles of the PRE-DISASTER Paradigm™ and DISASTER Paradigm™ to a potential real-life scenario.

Review the following scenario and answer the associated questions.

Scenario.   On August 24th, Tropical Storm James strengthens over the warm waters of the Atlantic Ocean into a category 3 hurricane. Sustained winds of 120 miles per hour are recorded, and a storm surge of 20 feet above normal is expected. The hurricane's diameter is nearly 400 miles, and the storm is moving forward at a rate of 16 miles per hour. A hurricane warning has been issued for the southern coast of your state, and the National Weather Service is predicting landfall in 4 days. The state governor and the governors of three neighboring states have declared states of emergency. Approximately 1 million people are expected to be affected by the storm, and the potential exists for hundreds of fatalities and thousands of injuries. As the storm moves closer to land, massive evacuations are required. Certain low-lying escape routes are already inundated by water 5 hours before the eye of the hurricane reaches land.

The National Hurricane Center and the Federal Emergency Management Agency (FEMA) hold numerous video teleconferences with state and federal emergency officials and provide them with the latest forecasts. As the storm approaches, state and local governments are given increasingly accurate forecasts and assessments of possible impacts. Federal and state emergency management officials preposition initial response resources outside the projected path of the storm.

On August 28th, Hurricane James makes landfall as a category 4 storm, striking the area and spawning tornadoes across central and southeastern portions of your state. A storm surge of 18 feet devastates the coastal plain with flooding, leaving 200,000 homes under water. Wind, water, and flying debris knock out electricity in most of the region, and the electric company expects it will take days to restore power. Rain associated with the storm causes rivers to overflow their banks, and several river systems are at record flood levels. Many people who were not able to or chose not to evacuate are trapped on the upper floors and roofs of their homes.

Temporary Red Cross shelters house 30,000 people on the edge of the disaster perimeter. Major hospitals in the area are severely damaged and flooded. Most were able to evacuate their critical patients before the storm hit but are now barely operational, running on emergency generators.

Initial assessments reveal that major portions of the affected region are flooded. Structures in low-lying areas were inundated when storm surges reached their peak. Many older facilities suffered structural collapse due to the swift influx of water and degradation of the supporting structural base. While newer facilities and structures survived the influx of water, many sustained heavy damage to contents on the lower levels. Nearly all shrubbery and trees in the storm's path were damaged or destroyed, generating massive amounts of debris. Debris was also generated from structures damaged or destroyed by the hurricane, as well as from numerous tornadoes spawned by the storm. Until the debris is cleared, rescue operations will be difficult because much of the area is reachable only by helicopters and boats. Wind and downed trees damaged nearly all of the electric transmission lines in the area. Most communications systems are not functioning because of damage and lack of power. Many structures will need to be demolished.

Temporary shelters throughout the region are filled to capacity. Hundreds of people are trapped and require search and rescue. The school year has just started, and there are 1300 school-aged children among the shelter residents. Thousands of citizens are homeless, and all affected communities are in serious need of drinking water. Food is in short supply and spoiling because of lack of refrigeration. Factories, chemical plants, sewage treatment plants, and other facilities in the region have suffered severe damage. Hundreds of thousands of gallons of extremely hazardous substances have spilled into the floodwaters. Gasoline, diesel fuel, and oil are leaking from underground storage tanks. A 95,000-ton tanker struck a bridge, breaching the hull of the vessel, which then began to leak oil into adjacent waters. Thousands of pets, domesticated animals, and wild animals have been killed or injured, and officials are overwhelmed with requests for assistance in finding lost pets. Health authorities are reporting an increased incidence of respiratory disease and anxiety-related disorders.

All transportation routes are damaged to some degree, and the port facility has also been adversely affected. Many businesses have experienced damage to buildings and infrastructure, as well as lost employees and customers. Military facilities are damaged, and assistance is needed for this community and to reconstitute these facilities. Local hospitals sustained severe damage, and those that are open are overwhelmed. Schools that are not severely damaged are being used as shelters for the disaster victims.

Event Summary

➤ *Casualties:* 1000 fatalities; 5000 injured victims requiring hospitalization

➤ *Infrastructure damage:* Numerous buildings destroyed; extensive amount of structural and vegetative debris; 200,000 homes destroyed

➤ *Evacuations/displaced persons:* 1 million evacuated; 150,000 seek shelter in safe areas

➤ *Economic impact:* Billions of dollars

Questions to Consider

Overview

1. Various agencies and professions have their own terminology when planning for and responding to a disaster. Considering this fact:

   ➤ What is the PRE-DISASTER Paradigm and why is it needed?

   ➤ What is the DISASTER Paradigm and why is it needed?

2. What are the elements of the PRE-DISASTER Paradigm? What specific issues are addressed by each element?

3. What are the elements of the DISASTER Paradigm? What specific issues are addressed by each element?

Preparation and Planning

4. What are the goals of disaster preparedness, and how do preparation and planning facilitate hurricane response and recovery efforts?

5. Discuss strategies for increasing individual and community resilience to this event.

Detection

6. What are the goals of detection and how does early detection, facilitate hurricane preparedness and response efforts?

7. What educational and informational resources are available to local health professionals and the public to help them prepare for, respond to, and recover from this event?

8. What health and safety information should be communicated to health care professionals and residents in affected areas?

Incident Management

9. What is the purpose of the National Incident Management System, or NIMS, during a hurricane?

10. What is the purpose and role of the incident command system during a hurricane?

11. What agencies would you expect to participate in the local incident command system? Who should be in charge?

Assess Hazards/Safety and Security

12. What are actual and potential hazards associated with this disaster?

13. What immediate health risks should be anticipated for responders and the affected population in the area? How will you and others protect against them?

14. What immediate safety risks should be anticipated for responders and the affected population in the area? How will you and others protect against them?

15. What immediate security risks should be anticipated for responders and the affected population in the area? How will you and others protect against them?

Support

16. What resources are available in the public and private sectors to assist with hurricane response efforts?

17. What level of government support can communities expect, and what should they be prepared to handle independently?

18. How is coordination among various agencies handled?

19. What opportunities are available for health professionals and non–health professionals to volunteer assistance?

Triage and Treatment

20. What is the goal of triage and treatment in a mass casualty emergency such as this hurricane scenario?

21. What are the public health implications of this disaster?

22. What types of injuries should health professionals be prepared to treat?

23. What health considerations are needed for persons in emergency shelters and for other displaced populations?

Evacuation

24. What is the purpose and primary goal of evacuation *before* landfall? What about evacuation *after* the hurricane hits?

25. What considerations are needed to evacuate elderly, immigrant, disabled, hospitalized, and incarcerated populations, children, and even pets? How would you deal with persons who refuse mandatory evacuation orders?

26. What items would you take along if forced to evacuate your home?

Recovery

27. What are the overall goals of recovery after a disaster?

28. When is recovery over?

29. What are some problems that might be encountered during the recovery period?

Conclusion

30. Is the PRE-DISASTER Paradigm useful to you in preparing for a hurricane scenario? Why or why not?

31. Is the DISASTER Paradigm useful to you in responding to a hurricane scenario? Why or why not?

HAZARDOUS MATERIALS RELEASE

Learning Objective. After completing this scenario, you will be able to apply the principles of the PRE-DISASTER Paradigm™ and DISASTER Paradigm™ to a potential real-life scenario.

Review the following scenario and answer the associated questions.

Scenario. On a humid, windy afternoon in July, a 98-car freight train rumbles toward your city (population 360,000) at 45 mph. The train, which has recently left a chemical processing district, carries tank cars containing several hazardous chemicals, among them propane and chlorine. Approximately 2 miles north of the city, a mechanical failure in the axle of one of the train cars causes that car and the 30 immediately behind it to derail. The wreckage includes 10 propane tank cars and six chlorine tank cars.

You witness the derailment and decide to help. Other bystanders have already called 911, but emergency responders are delayed because of traffic and crowd congestion. You consider entering the scene to assist.

Fire department and law enforcement personnel, as well as the local hazardous materials (HAZMAT) team, arrive and implement an incident command system. Intermittent explosions rock the scene as propane tanks in the wreckage ignite.

The derailment occurs next to a busy two-lane highway. Sixteen automobiles, including a school bus, sustain significant damage from flying debris and collisions with other vehicles. At least 60 people need immediate onsite assistance. The HAZMAT team has established that all of the derailed chlorine tank cars have ruptured and are leaking gas into the air. Numerous propane tanks have exploded, and several more are in danger of igniting.

Nearby hospitals have been alerted about the incident and are preparing to receive an influx of casualties. Located immediately adjacent to the accident site are a 150-unit mobile home park, an elementary school with 200 students, and three small manufacturing businesses with approximately 20 employees each. A busy state highway runs just south of the tracks, and a small road crosses the tracks just ahead of the accident scene. A river flows 4 miles to the south. As many as 700,000 people may be at risk of exposure as the gas plume moves downwind (which could extend as far as 25 miles). Residents in the affected and adjacent communities are calling their physicians and local public health authorities for information and instructions to protect themselves and their families.

Event Summary

➤ *Casualties:* At least 60 casualties at the scene; thousands of community residents are at risk.

➤ *Infrastructure damage:* There may be significant damage to the railway. Decontamination of waterways may present a major challenge as well.

Any local waterways or wetlands will absorb the chlorine gas, creating hydrochloric acid and increasing the acidity (lowering the pH) of the water. Environmental effects, especially public safety concerns, are likely to significantly delay rebuilding efforts. Decontamination, destruction, disposal, and replacement costs could reach millions of dollars. The local economy will be affected by public apprehension. Significant disruptions in health care will occur because of the overwhelming demand of the injured and the "worried well."

➤ *Evacuations/displaced persons:* Evacuation/sheltering/protection of downwind populations will be required. Evacuation could become chaotic if panic-stricken residents attempt to flee the area. Coordinated efforts will be needed to manage evacuations (whether ordered or spontaneous), protect vulnerable populations, establish temporary sheltering alternatives and interim housing, and provide food for evacuees.

➤ *Economic impact:* Millions of dollars

Questions to Consider

Overview

1. Various agencies and professions have their own terminology when planning for and responding to a disaster. Considering this fact:

   ➤ What is the PRE-DISASTER Paradigm and why is it needed?

   ➤ What is the DISASTER Paradigm and why is it needed?

2. What are the elements of the PRE-DISASTER Paradigm? What specific issues are addressed by each element?

3. What are the elements of the DISASTER Paradigm? What specific issues are addressed by each element?

Preparation and Planning

4. What are the goals of disaster preparedness, and how do preparation and planning facilitate local response and recovery efforts?

5. Discuss strategies for increasing individual and community resilience to this event.

Detection

6. You witness the derailment and decide to help. What would you do? Discuss immediate considerations that should guide your initial response. Prioritize your actions.

7. What educational and informational resources are available to local health professionals and the public to help them prepare for, respond to, and recover from this event?

8. What health and safety information should be communicated to health care professionals and residents in the surrounding area?

Incident Management

9. What is the purpose of the National Incident Management System, or NIMS, during this event?

10. What is the purpose and role of the incident command system?

11. What agencies would you expect to participate in the local incident command system? Who should be in charge?

Assess Hazards/Safety and Security

12. What are the actual and potential hazards associated with this event?

13. What immediate health risks should be anticipated for responders and the affected population? How will you and others protect against them?

14. What immediate safety risks should be anticipated for responders and the affected population? How will you and others protect against them?

15. What immediate security risks should be anticipated for responders and the affected population? How will you and others protect against them?

Support

16. What resources are available in the public and private sectors to assist with response efforts?

17. What level of government support can communities expect, and what should they be prepared to handle independently?

18. How is coordination among various agencies handled?

Triage and Treatment

19. What is the purpose of mass casualty triage at the scene? Where would you implement such a system?

20. What are the public health implications of this disaster?

21. What types of injuries would you expect to see at the scene?

22. What might constitute appropriate treatment at the scene?

Evacuation

23. What is the purpose and primary goal of evacuation from the scene?

24. What are the risks of evacuating local residents?

25. What considerations are needed to evacuate elderly, immigrant, disabled, hospitalized, and incarcerated populations, children, and even pets? How would you deal with persons who refuse mandatory evacuation orders?

26. What items would you take along if forced to evacuate your home?

Recovery

27. What are the overall goals of recovery in this scenario?

28. What are some problems that might be encountered during the recovery period?

Conclusion

29. Is the PRE-DISASTER Paradigm useful to you in preparing for a hazardous materials release scenario? Why or why not?

30. Is the DISASTER Paradigm useful to you in responding to a hazardous materials release scenario? Why or why not?

INFLUENZA PANDEMIC

Learning Objective.   After completing this scenario, you will be able to apply the principles of the PRE-DISASTER Paradigm™ and DISASTER Paradigm™ to a potential real-life scenario.

Review the following scenario and answer the associated questions.

Scenario.   *Day 1:* You are a health professional in a small city (population 75,000). Recently, you joined the local Medical Reserve Corps (MRC) unit and have just completed training. During a monthly MRC meeting at the community center, your group is distracted by a breaking news report that appears on the television screen:

> *Hospitals throughout Southeast Asia are being overwhelmed by a potentially lethal flu-like illness. Health authorities in Hong Kong and Singapore are considering quarantine measures to control the spread of this disease. The illness appears to have a mortality rate of 30% and affects persons of all ages. Available vaccines seem to provide no protection. Researchers are working around the clock to determine the effectiveness of other treatments in controlling this outbreak.*

You discuss the implications of this news with your team and agree to stay in close communication. Your team agrees to meet in 3 days to discuss further developments.

Day 3: Your MRC unit reconvenes at the community center and reflects on the news of the past 72 hours. Today, you receive word that disease outbreaks have been reported in Europe, Canada, and the United States. Twelve suspected cases of the disease have been reported in two neighboring states.

The World Health Organization (WHO) and the Centers for Disease Control and Prevention (CDC) have determined that the outbreak is due to a novel influenza A virus, which has the capacity for efficient and sustained human-to-human transmission in the general population. Both agencies have declared that a global influenza pandemic is in progress. China, Taiwan, Singapore, and Indonesia have imposed strict travel restrictions, and many other countries are taking similar actions. Standard case definitions have been transmitted to all US health care facilities and public health agencies via the CDC Health Alert Network.

Government officials in your community have called an emergency meeting of local public health, hospital, emergency medical services, public safety, emergency management, business, and community leaders to discuss activation of the local pandemic influenza plan.

Day 7: The state health department has issued an urgent medical bulletin to all health professionals and facilities in the state notifying them that 20 cases of the novel influenza virus have been confirmed in your state; three of these occurred in your county. On the basis of limited data from the WHO and the CDC, it appears that an experimental drug may be effective in treating this disease. No vaccine is available and it may take up to a year before one can be developed. Your MRC unit has been placed on alert, and you have been asked to prepare for possible deployment.

Day 12: Your MRC unit has been deployed to the local high school gymnasium to function as a point of distribution (POD) prophylaxis dispensing site for limited quantities of the antiviral drug that have been made available to your community. Outside the gymnasium, police are being confronted by a growing crowd of persons seeking medical attention and treatment.

Day 15: The high school gymnasium has been converted from a POD prophylaxis dispensing site into an alternate care site. A continuous stream of patients with respiratory symptoms consistent with novel influenza infection flows into the gymnasium, other alternate care sites, and local emergency departments. You are now being asked to assist with the assessment and care of 150 patients (110 adults, 40 children) with respiratory symptoms suggestive of novel influenza. Treatment is limited to comfort and supportive care.

➤ Fifteen patients (11 adults, four children) need advanced respiratory care and await transport to local hospitals.

➤ A number of patients have additional medical problems such as hypertension, diabetes, asthma, and heart disease.

➤ It has been about 72 hours since you and your group have been activated in response to the rising pandemic.

➤ While you have been asked to remain at the gymnasium until further notice, you have been there for 3 days now, away from family and loved ones.

Day 60: The first wave of the pandemic continues for the next 2 months. While no new cases have been reported in your state during the past 2 weeks, 20 new cases of novel influenza have been just been reported in a neighboring state.

Questions to Consider

Overview

1. Various agencies and professions have their own terminology when planning for and responding to a disaster. Considering this fact,

  ➤ What is the PRE-DISASTER Paradigm and why is it needed?

  ➤ What is the DISASTER Paradigm and why is it needed?

2. What are the elements of the PRE-DISASTER Paradigm? What specific issues are addressed by each element?

3. What are the elements of the DISASTER Paradigm? What specific issues are addressed by each element?

Preparation and Planning

4. What are the goals of public health preparedness, and how do preparation and planning facilitate pandemic response and recovery efforts?

5. Discuss strategies for increasing individual and community resilience to this event.

Detection

6. What are the goals of detection in a pandemic and how does early detection facilitate preparedness and response efforts?

7. What is the function and role of the public health system in an infectious disease outbreak?

8. What educational and informational resources are available to local health professionals and the public to help them prepare for, respond to, and recover from this event?

9. What health information should be communicated to health care professionals and community residents?

Incident Management

10. What is the purpose of the National Incident Management System, or NIMS, during a pandemic?

11. What is the purpose and role of the incident command system during a pandemic? Who should be in charge?

Assess Hazards/Safety and Security

12. What are the immediate health concerns for first responders and local citizens?

13. What are the immediate safety concerns for first responders and local citizens?

14. What are the immediate security concerns for first responders and local citizens?

Support

15. What are your expectations for public and private sector support in managing this outbreak?

16. What opportunities are available for health professionals and non–health professionals to volunteer assistance?

Triage and Treatment

17. What is the goal of triage and treatment in a pandemic?

18. What actions can you take to protect yourself from exposure to the pandemic virus?

19. What actions can your community take to protect citizens from exposure to the pandemic virus?

20. How would you deal with people who refuse mandatory vaccination or quarantine orders?

Evacuation

21. What items should be stockpiled in advance if you need to be confined at home for an extended period of time?

22. Many volunteers (you included) have been working long hours at the alternative care facility (high school gymnasium) and want to leave to be with loved ones and families. Is this acceptable, and if so, how could this best be accommodated?

Recovery

23. What are the overall goals of recovery after a pandemic?

24. When can influenza control measures be relaxed? Who makes these decisions?

Conclusion

25. Is the PRE-DISASTER Paradigm useful to you in preparing for an influenza pandemic scenario? Why or why not?

26. Is the DISASTER Paradigm useful to you in responding to an influenza pandemic scenario? Why or why not?

TERRORIST BOMBING

Learning Objective.   After completing this scenario, you will be able to apply the principles of the PRE-DISASTER Paradigm™ and DISASTER Paradigm™ to a potential real-life scenario.

Review the following scenario and answer the associated questions.

Scenario.   During a professional baseball game (with almost 55,000 spectators), several small explosive devices hidden at various points throughout the stadium are detonated simultaneously via remote control transmitters. About 20 individuals sustain minor injuries from flying debris. Chaos ensues as the crowd flees to the exits. Many run to their cars, which are parked in an adjacent underground garage filled to capacity. Others rush to the main street outside the stadium, which is a major bus route for the city. The stadium is located in a densely populated, downtown urban environment.

Two sport utility vehicles (SUVs) have been outfitted as large vehicle bombs. One has been parked for hours in the underground garage; the other was parked minutes ago on the main street outside the stadium, next to the main bus stop. Each SUV carries about 3000 pounds of a readily attainable, conventional explosive. The vehicle bombs are remotely detonated, approximately 15 minutes after the initial stadium blasts, when both the garage and the street are filled with frantic people attempting to escape the area.

Driving past the stadium, you witness the vehicle bomb explosions and decide to help. Other bystanders have already called 911, but emergency responders are delayed because of traffic and crowd congestion. You consider running into the parking garage to assist. Although you are not a licensed health professional, you have been trained in Core Disaster Life Support.

Emergency response personnel begin to arrive at the scene within minutes of the explosions. Medical responders initiate assessment, triage, and emergency treatment of injured persons. It is determined that 120 fatalities occurred in the parking garage and 80 on the street; at least 500 persons sustained injuries that require medical attention. Multiple ambulances and helicopters arrive at the scene to begin evacuation of the most critically injured victims. Nearby hospitals are alerted that at least 70 patients will be leaving the scene within the hour.

Event Summary

➤ *Casualties:* 200 fatalities; 500 victims may require hospitalization

➤ *Infrastructure damage:* Structures affected by blast and fire

➤ *Evacuations/displaced persons:* Evacuation of immediate area around the explosion results in approximately 1000 people seeking shelter in safe areas

➤ *Economic Impact:* Millions of dollars

Questions to Consider

Overview

1. Various agencies and professions have their own terminology when planning for and responding to a disaster. Considering this fact:

   ➤ What is the PRE-DISASTER Paradigm and why is it needed?

   ➤ What is the DISASTER Paradigm and why is it needed?

2. What are the elements of the PRE-DISASTER Paradigm? What specific issues are addressed by each element?

3. What are the elements of the DISASTER Paradigm? What specific issues are addressed by each element?

Preparation and Planning

4. What are the goals of disaster preparedness, and how do preparation and planning facilitate response and recovery efforts to this terrorist event?

5. Discuss strategies for increasing individual and community resilience to this event.

Detection

6. You witness the bombing outside the stadium and decide to help. What would you do? Discuss immediate considerations that should guide your initial response. Prioritize your actions.

7. What educational and informational resources are available to local health professionals and the public to help them prepare for, respond to, and recover from this event?

8. What health and safety information should be communicated to health care professionals and residents in the surrounding area?

Incident Management

9. What is the purpose of the National Incident Management System, or NIMS, during this event?

10. What is the purpose and role of the incident command system?

11. What agencies would you expect to participate in the incident command system? Who should be in charge?

Assess Hazards/Safety and Security

12. What are the actual and potential hazards associated with this event?

13. What immediate health risks should be anticipated for responders and the affected population in the parking garage and on the street? How will you and others protect against them?

14. What immediate safety risks should be anticipated for responders and the affected population in the parking garage and on the street? How will you and others protect against them?

15. What immediate security risks should be anticipated for responders and the affected population in the parking garage and on the street? How will you and others protect against them?

Support

16. What resources are available in the public and private sectors to assist with response efforts?

17. What level of government support can communities expect, and what should they be prepared to handle independently?

18. How is coordination among various agencies handled?

Triage and Treatment

19. What is the purpose of mass casualty triage at the scene?

20. What types of injuries are most likely to be seen in persons who were in the stadium, in the parking garage, and on the street outside the stadium? Would you expect the pattern of injuries to be identical for these situations?

21. What are the public health implications of this disaster?

22. What might constitute appropriate treatment at the scene?

Evacuation

23. What is the purpose and primary goal of evacuation from the scene?

24. What are the risks of evacuating local residents?

25. What considerations are needed to evacuate elderly, immigrant, disabled, hospitalized, and incarcerated populations, children, and even pets? How would you deal with persons who refuse mandatory evacuation orders?

26. What items would you take along if forced to evacuate your home?

Recovery

27. What are the overall goals of recovery in a disaster?

28. What are some problems that might be encountered during the recovery period?

Conclusion

29. Is the PRE-DISASTER Paradigm useful to you in preparing for a terrorist bombing scenario? Why or why not?

30. Is the DISASTER Paradigm useful to you in responding to a terrorist bombing scenario? Why or why not?

SCENARIO DEBRIEF AND CONTENT EVALUATION

After completing the self-learning scenarios, please answer the following questions and send a copy of the completed form to the NDLS™ Program Office; 515 North State Street, Chicago, IL 60654; or fax a copy to 312 464-5841. An electronic version of this form also can be found under "CDLS® Course Information" at http://www.NDLSF.org. Your feedback is appreciated and will be considered in further revisions of the CDLS course and course manual.

1. Did the PRE-DISASTER Paradigm™ help you recall the information required to answer the scenario questions?

2. Did the DISASTER Paradigm™ help you recall the information required to answer the scenario questions?

3. Does the PRE-DISASTER Paradigm help you remember information about disaster preparedness in general?

4. Does the DISASTER Paradigm help you remember information about responding to disasters in general?

5. Did the CDLS course and course manual help you in thinking through these "real-life" disaster scenarios?

6. Were the self-learning scenarios useful in helping reinforce material presented in the CDLS course and course manual?

7. What was and was not included in the CDLS course and course manual that was relevant to the scenario-based questions?

8. Did anything come up during the self-learning scenarios that you thought would be important information to know in a real disaster that was not covered in the CDLS course or course manual?

9. Many health professionals and first responders think that a consequence of their job is that they are often put in dangerous situations. Do you think CDLS course content has changed the way you view how to protect yourself in a disaster?

10. Did you understand the role of the health system in a disaster situation before taking the CDLS course and reading this course manual? Do you have a better understanding of the health system after taking this course? If so, how?

Emergency Notification Form

EMERGENCY NOTIFICATION FORM

Ambulance (local emergency medical dispatch number) _____

Police department _____

Fire department _____

Local poison control center _____

Local health department _____

State health department _____

Hospital emergency department _____

Physician _____

Physician _____

Psychiatrist or other mental health professional _____

24-hour pharmacy _____

Other neighborhood pharmacy _____

Health insurance number _____

Work number _____

Work number _____

Dentist _____

Babysitter _____

School _____

School _____

Day care center _____

Veterinarian _____

Electric company _____

Gas company _____

Water company _____

Neighbor _____

Neighbor _____

Relative _____

Relative _____

Other _____

_____

CDLS® Quick Reference Guide

PRE-DISASTER Paradigm™		
P	Planning and Practice	Do your community and workplace have disaster plans? Do you have a personal or family plan? Are these plans practiced and evaluated regularly?
R	Resilience	What measures are in place to help individuals and communities cope with physical and psychological trauma?
E	Education	Are opportunities available for competency-based education and training in disaster medicine and public health preparedness to meet the needs of all health professionals?

DISASTER Paradigm™		
D	Detect	Do needs exceed resources? Contact appropriate authorities and agencies.
I	Incident Management	What is your role? Who is the incident commander?
S	Scene Safety/Security	Is the scene secure? Is it safe to enter?
A	Assess Hazards	Fire? Hazardous materials? Radiation? Building collapse? Downed power lines? Secondary devices?
S	Support	What outside assistance is needed (eg, police, fire, emergency medical services, government, other)? Can adequate surge capability and capacity be established to meet local public safety/health needs and priorities?
T	Triage and Treatment	Are protocols, procedures, and resources in place for the rapid triage and immediate treatment of casualties? What public health interventions are needed?
E	Evacuation	Are enough transport units in route to the scene? Should affected persons evacuate or shelter-in-place?
R	Recovery	Has critical infrastructure been damaged? What are the short- and long-term health needs of affected individuals and communities?

ABCs of Scene Safety and Hazard Assessment

<u>A</u>   Assess hazards (situational awareness of all hazards, primary and secondary)

<u>B</u>   Barriers in place to protect public health, safety, and security (personal protective equipment; time, distance, shielding; control of scene entry and exit)

<u>C</u>   Communicate (call 911; inform incident commander; involve media)

Essential First Aid Skills for All Health System Responders

➤ Scene and casualty assessment

➤ Resuscitation

➤ Control of bleeding and treatment of shock

➤ Management of fractures and dislocations

➤ Care of the unconscious casualty

➤ Safe movement of injured persons

CDLS® Quick Reference Sheets

Disaster Preparedness Steps for All Citizens

Key Action Steps in a Natural Disaster

Key Points About Biologic Emergencies

Key Points About Bombings

Key Points About Chemical Emergencies

Key Points About Radiation Emergencies

Key Points to Help Cope with Disaster

CDLS QUICK REFERENCE SHEETS

CDLS Tip Sheet: Disaster Preparedness Steps for All Citizens

➤ Understand the disaster risks in your community. Ask local authorities about possible hazards that may affect your community and what the risks might be for you and your family.

➤ Prepare and practice an emergency plan with your family.

➤ Prepare a disaster supply kit.

➤ Be aware of your surroundings, and trust your instincts. If something does not seem right, it probably isn't.

➤ Take precautions when traveling. Be aware of conspicuous or unusual behavior. Do not accept packages from strangers. Do not leave luggage unattended. Learn where emergency exits are located in buildings you frequent.

➤ Promptly report unusual behavior, suspicious or unattended packages, and strange devices to law enforcement or security personnel.

➤ Learn about emergency preparedness and response plans for your community, schools, and place of employment. Know the location of these plans. Participate in local disaster drills and exercises as appropriate.

➤ Learn about your community's emergency warning system and emergency communication plan.

➤ Know how to contact local medical, public health, and law enforcement authorities.

➤ Be aware of available medical and mental health information and resources and how to access them immediately and in various ways.

➤ Be prepared emotionally; understand stress and how to deal with it.

➤ Be prepared physically; maintain a healthy lifestyle. Eat a well-balanced diet, be physically active, get adequate sleep, and avoid tobacco, alcohol, and other drugs.

➤ Learn immediate actions to protect your health and safety, as well as that of your family and your neighbors.

➤ Take measures to protect your home and personal belongings; be sure to have working fire extinguishers, smoke detectors, and carbon monoxide detectors.

➤ Learn first aid and basic life support procedures; participate in additional education and training programs to improve your knowledge, ability, and willingness to respond to an emergency or mass casualty situation.

➤ Learn about local disaster relief services that can provide assistance. Contact local agencies and organizations about volunteer opportunities.

CDLS Tip Sheet: Key Action Steps in a Natural Disaster

➤ Stay tuned to the local emergency response network or news station for up-to-date information and instructions.

➤ If you were evacuated, return home only after local officials tell you it is safe.

➤ Stay away from floodwaters. Do not drive or walk through flowing floodwaters!

➤ Check yourself and family members for injuries. Help those who may need special assistance and give first aid where appropriate.

➤ Avoid loose or dangling power lines, and report them to the power company, police, or fire department.

➤ Enter your home or any building with caution. Do not enter if there is water around the building.

➤ Use flashlights to examine walls, floors, doors, staircases, and windows. Consider calling a qualified person to inspect foundations for cracks and make sure the building is not in danger of collapsing.

➤ Look for fire hazards such as flooded electrical circuits or submerged furnaces and appliances.

➤ Check for gas leaks. If you smell gas or hear a hissing noise, open a window and leave quickly. Turn off the gas at the outside main valve, and call the gas company from a neighbor's home.

➤ Look for electrical system damage. If you see sparks or frayed wires, turn off the electricity at the main fuse box or circuit breaker. Do not step in water to get to the fuse box or circuit breaker before calling an electrician for advice.

➤ Check for sewage and water line damage. If you think sewage lines are damaged, don't use toilets, and call a plumber. If water pipes are damaged, don't use tap water, and call the water company.

➤ Watch out for animals, especially poisonous snakes that may have entered the building with floodwaters.

➤ Take pictures of the damage for insurance claims.

➤ Avoid drinking or preparing food with tap water until local officials tell you it is not contaminated.

➤ Open windows and doors to ventilate and dry out your home.

➤ Telephone systems may be jammed. Use the telephone for emergency calls only.

CDLS Tip Sheet: Key Points About Biologic Emergencies

➤ Effective response to an infectious disease outbreak depends on individual clinicians (who well may be the "first responders") having the knowledge and necessary level of awareness to suspect that something unusual might be occurring and then to activate the public health system.

➤ Health professionals should report noticeable increases in unusual illnesses, symptom complexes, or disease patterns (even without definitive diagnosis) to public health authorities.

➤ Prompt reporting of unusual patterns of illness can allow public health officials to initiate an epidemiologic investigation earlier than would be possible if the report awaited definitive etiologic diagnosis.

➤ Some biologic agents (for example, anthrax spores) can survive in the environment for long periods, creating a long-term hazard.

➤ The start of a biologic emergency may be difficult to detect. For some infectious agents, the disease may spread for weeks before it is detected.

➤ The severity of a biologic emergency will vary depending on the type of agent, its virulence, the route of exposure, and susceptibility of the victim to infection.

➤ Unlike nuclear, chemical, and explosive events, the onset of a biologic emergency will probably be insidious. A contagious biologic agent has the potential for large-scale spread before detection (which is dependent on traditional disease surveillance methods).

➤ In a biologic emergency, public health officials may not immediately be able to provide complete information on appropriate personal and community actions to limit disease spread. It will take time to determine what the illness is, how it should be treated, and who is in danger. It is important to listen to television, radio, or emergency alert systems for up-to-date information and instructions.

➤ Local or state health officials will monitor the situation and recommend protective action. They will let you know what symptoms to look for, areas in danger, if medications or vaccinations are being distributed, and where to seek medical attention. The most appropriate action will depend on the situation.

➤ Some biologic agents may be spread easily from infected persons to others. Health officials will provide clearly defined instructions for dealing with exposed or infected persons.

➤ Infection control precautions must be used until thorough assessment has been performed or the specific biologic agent is identified. Health professionals must first protect themselves (eg, by using the appropriate PPE) to minimize exposure.

➤ For some infectious agents, secondary and tertiary transmission may continue for weeks or months after the initial outbreak. This requires that medical treatment facilities have clearly defined procedures for handling infected casualties, many of whom will transport themselves to the facility.

➤ In an epidemic, overwhelming numbers of critically ill patients will require acute and follow-up medical care. Both infected persons and persons who fear they may have been exposed (the "well but worried") will seek medical attention, with a corresponding need for medical consultation, medical supplies, diagnostic tests, and hospital beds.

IMPORTANT CLUES THAT MAY SIGNAL A BIOLOGIC EMERGENCY

➤ A single suspected case of an uncommon disease

➤ Single or multiple cases of a suspected common disease or syndrome that does not respond to treatment as expected

➤ Clusters of a similar illness occurring in the same time frame in different locales

➤ Unusual clinical, geographic, seasonal, or temporal presentation of a disease and/or unusual transmission route

➤ Unexplained increase in incidence of an endemic disease

➤ Unusual illness that affects a large, disparate population or is unusual for a population or age group

➤ Unusual pattern of illness or death among animals or humans

➤ Sudden increase in the following nonspecific illnesses:

- Pneumonia, influenza-like illness, or fever with atypical features

- Bleeding disorders

- Unexplained rashes and mucosal or skin irritation, particularly in adults

- Neuromuscular illness, such as muscle weakness and paralysis

- Diarrhea

CDLS Tip Sheet: Key Points About Bombings

➤ Severely injured victims may bypass triage at the disaster scene and go directly to the closest hospitals.

➤ Bombs and explosions can cause unique patterns of injury, involving multiple organs. In the United States, such injuries are seldom seen outside of military combat.

➤ Predominant injuries involve multiple penetrating injuries and blunt trauma.

➤ Explosions in confined spaces (buildings, large vehicles, mines) and/or structural collapse are associated with greater morbidity and mortality.

➤ Primary blast injuries in survivors are predominantly seen in confined-space explosions.

➤ Time is critical in the treatment of blast injury; repeatedly examine and assess affected patients. It is important for health care professionals to become familiar with pathophysiology, diagnosis, and treatment considerations for traumatic brain injury in advance of an explosive event.

➤ All bombing events may result in chemical and/or radiologic contamination of people and surrounding environments. Medical help should never be delayed because of the possibility of radioactive contamination of the person. The use of standard protective measures is effective in protecting first responders and other caregivers against contamination with radioactive materials.

➤ The effects of an explosion depend on the amount of explosive materials used and how the device was made, the surrounding environment, the delivery method, and the distance and barriers between the victim and the blast.

➤ People who were near an explosion should receive follow-up medical examinations. Some health effects may be delayed.

➤ After a bombing or other explosion, local authorities will monitor the situation and recommend protective action. The most appropriate action will depend on the situation. It is important to listen to television, radio, or emergency alert systems for up-to-date information and instructions. People may be advised to "shelter-in-place," which means to stay at home or at work, or to move to another location.

CDLS Tip Sheet: Key Points About Chemical Emergencies

➤ Evaluate chemical risks in the community by using information from the Local Emergency Planning Committee and local emergency management office. Determine proximity to factories, highways, or railroads that may produce or transport potentially hazardous chemicals.

➤ Learn about community plans for responding to hazardous materials incidents at an industrial plant or other facility or a transportation incident involving hazardous materials.

➤ Primary detection of exposure to chemical agents is based on the signs and symptoms in exposed persons.

➤ The release of a chemical agent may be difficult to identify easily:

- Symptoms of exposure to some chemical agents can be similar to those of common diseases, such as gastroenteritis (stomach flu).

- Immediate symptoms of certain chemical exposures might be nonexistent or mild despite the risk for long-term effects.

- Health care professionals may be less familiar with illnesses suggesting exposure to chemical agents than with illnesses they treat more frequently.

➤ Confirmation of a chemical agent, using detection equipment or laboratory analyses, will take time and will not likely contribute to immediate casualty management.

➤ Treating exposed persons by clinical syndrome rather than by specific agent probably is the most pragmatic approach to the treatment of illness caused by chemical exposures.

➤ After the release of a chemical agent, local authorities will monitor the situation and recommend protective action. The most appropriate action will depend on the situation. It is important to listen to television, radio, or emergency alert systems for up-to-date information and instructions. People may be advised to "shelter-in-place," which means to stay at home or at work, or to move to another location.

➤ If instructed to remain at home or at work, people should:

- Close doors and windows and turn off all ventilation, including furnaces, air conditioners, vents, and fans.

- Seek shelter in an internal room and take their disaster supply kit.

➤ If caught outside during a chemical incident, people should try to stay uphill and upwind of the scene. Hazardous gases and mists are generally heavier than air and can be transported quickly by the wind.

➤ Effects from exposure to chemical agents will vary depending on the:

- Type of agent

- Route of exposure (skin, inhaled, ingested)

- Amount and strength of the chemical

- Duration of exposure

- Preexisting medical conditions (for example, people with heart or respiratory diseases)

➤ Precautions (eg, use of personal protective gear and decontamination) must be utilized by first responders to avoid contaminating themselves and other emergency personnel, as well as transport vehicles and treatment facilities.

(continued)

➤ Clothing should be removed, and skin should be washed with soap and large amounts of water to remove external chemical contamination.

➤ It is likely that many people will arrive at hospitals by private vehicle without proper decontamination.

➤ Stress on patients and providers will cause further confusion; the potential for mass hysteria is high.

IMPORTANT CLUES THAT MAY SUGGEST A CHEMICAL EMERGENCY

➤ An unusual increase in the number of patients seeking care for a rapid onset of symptoms after exposure to a potentially contaminated medium (eg, paresthesias and vomiting within minutes of eating a meal)

➤ Rapid onset of illness with little or no warning

➤ Unexplained illness or death among young or previously healthy persons

➤ Presence of an unexplained odor, low-level clouds, or vapors at the scene

➤ Emission of unexplained odors by patients

➤ Clusters of illness in persons who have common characteristics, such as drinking water from the same source

➤ Unexplained death of plants, fish, or animals (domestic or wild)

➤ A syndrome (ie, a constellation of clinical signs and symptoms in patients) suggesting a disease associated commonly with a known chemical exposure:

  – Sudden unexplained weakness, collapse, apnea, or convulsions in previously healthy persons

  – Dimmed or blurred vision

  – Hypersecretion syndromes (eg, tearing, drooling, diarrhea)

  – Inhalation syndromes (eye, nose, throat, chest irritation; shortness of breath)

  – Burn-like syndromes (redness, blistering, itching, sloughing)

CDLS Tip Sheet: Key Points About Radiation Emergencies

➤ Although the likelihood of a thermonuclear war is low, the possibility of either a single nuclear detonation or an incident involving unintentional or deliberate radiologic contamination has increased; the most likely deliberate radiation event involves direct placement of a radioactive source in a public place or detonation of a high-yield explosive contaminated with radioactive material (ie, a "dirty bomb").

➤ The primary risk of a dirty bomb or other isolated radiation incident is the psychological impact on a population rather than acute or delayed radiation sickness.

➤ The most appropriate action will depend on the situation. People should stay tuned to the local emergency response network or news stations for up-to-date information and instructions.

➤ After a release of radioactive materials, local authorities will monitor the levels of radiation and determine what protective actions to take. If a radiation emergency involves the release of large amounts of radioactive materials, people may be advised to "shelter-in-place," which means to stay in at home or at work, or to move to another location.

➤ If instructed to remain at home or at work, people should:

– Close doors and windows and turn off all ventilation, including furnaces, air conditioners, vents, and fans

– Seek shelter in an internal room and take their disaster supply kit

➤ The longer one is exposed to radiation, the greater the dose; casualties should be removed from the disaster scene as quickly as possible.

➤ Radiation exposure is inversely related to the square of the distance from the source; the farther away a person is from the source, the lower the radiation dose.

➤ Heavy-density materials such as lead and concrete are best for shielding from gamma rays and X-rays; plastics are preferred for shielding beta particles. Water and concrete are used as shielding material for neutrons. Overall, concrete and earth are the most effective shielding materials.

➤ When caring for radiation casualties, primary consideration should be given to:

– Addressing immediate critical care needs (eg, traumatic injuries, burns)

– Eliminating additional radiation risk to the patient

– Preventing contamination and radiation exposure of first responders and health care workers

➤ Emergency responders should wear protective gloves, protective clothing, and radiation dosimeters; respirators or protective masks can prevent inhalation of radioactive particles.

➤ Removal of clothing and washing with soap and copious amounts of water are sufficient to remove most external radiation contamination.

➤ Life-threatening injuries should be treated first. Radiation treatment, other than decontamination, is a secondary concern; most deaths from radiation occur as a result of bone marrow damage and secondary infection.

➤ People being examined for potential radiation exposure may not exhibit significant symptoms when first examined (even if they received a considerable radiation dose) because of the characteristic delayed onset of symptoms after exposure. Follow-up examination during the ensuing hours and days is essential to establish the true nature and extent of exposure.

(continued)

➤ Any externally contaminated casualty without respiratory protection should be evaluated for internal contamination.

➤ Documentation of clinical signs and symptoms (affecting the hematopoietic, gastrointestinal, cerebrovascular, and cutaneous systems) over time is essential for triage of casualties, selection of therapy, and assignment of prognosis.

➤ The health effects of radiation exposure are directly related to the amount of radiation absorbed by the body (radiation dose) and are determined by the:

 – Radiation type (alpha, beta, X-rays, or gamma radiation)

 – Means of exposure, internal or external (absorbed by the skin, inhaled, or ingested)

 – Length of time exposed

➤ Determination of radiation exposure is expedited by the evaluation of various blood components (eg, lympho-cytopenia) and time of onset of the prodromal syndrome (eg, nausea, vomiting, anorexia).

➤ Patients with severe radiation exposure develop burns that are subject to secondary infection; antiseptic wound care is critical.

➤ Possible pharmaceutical countermeasures to ionizing radiation can be categorized broadly into three groups:

 – Drugs that prevent initial radiation injury

 – Drugs that repair the molecular damage caused by radiation

 – Drugs that stimulate proliferation of surviving stem and progenitor cells

➤ The decision to use oral and intravenous drugs for internally contaminated patients should be made after consultation with a nuclear medicine physician or other radiation therapy specialist.

➤ Bone marrow suppression associated with high-dose radiation exposures requires sophisticated treatment such as transfusion of blood products and use of colony-stimulating growth factors and cytokines along with antimicrobial therapy and immunosuppression precautions as the risk of infection and hemorrhaging develops.

➤ When there is concern about a known or suspected exposure to radioactive iodine (eg, nuclear power plant incident), potassium iodide (KI) should be administered empirically as a thyroid blocking agent. KI will not protect a person from other radioactive materials or protect other parts of the body from radiation exposure. A one-time dose at levels recommended by the Food and Drug Administration (FDA) is usually all that is required. Current FDA recommendations are as follows:

 – Because KI is effective for only about 24 hours, it can be administered daily until the exposure risk is eliminated

 – If possible, at-risk children should receive KI before exposure or immediately afterward

 – Women who are breastfeeding should take the adult KI dose; the infant should receive the recommended infant dose

CDLS Tip Sheet: Key Points to Help Cope with Disaster

➤ Provide basic resources including food, shelter, communication, transportation, information, guidance, and medical and mental health services for victims and responders.

➤ Create a local infrastructure to address the mental health needs of children and their families in times of disaster or crisis; this includes interventions and programs to promote individual and community resilience and prevent adverse psychological effects.

➤ Implement surveillance systems for psychological consequences, including distress responses, behavior changes, and psychiatric illness, and markers of individual and community functioning before, during, and after a disaster or other traumatic event.

➤ Screen for psychological symptoms at the individual level.

➤ Provide for treatment of acute and long-term effects of trauma.

➤ Provide resources for longer-term general human service needs that contribute to psychological functioning (eg, housing, financial assistance when the event creates job loss).

➤ Develop effective risk communication protocols for the dissemination of information to the public, the media political leaders, and service providers.

➤ Train service providers (in medical, public health, emergency management, and mental health systems) to respond to disasters and to protect themselves against psychological trauma.

➤ Review local and regional capacity to handle a large increase in demand for services to address psychological consequences in the event of a disaster or public health emergency.

➤ Integrate case-finding ability to locate individuals who have not utilized mental health services but need them, including underserved, marginalized, and unrecognized groups of people (eg, undocumented immigrants, homebound persons, and others with unidentified needs).

➤ Educate yourself about the potential danger. Keep informed about breaking news and developments. If television or other news reports greatly increase your feelings of anxiety and helplessness, avoid them; you don't need every graphic detail.

➤ Avoid overexposure to news rebroadcasts of the events. Television news of traumatic events can be particularly frightening to children, especially when it is viewed repeatedly.

➤ Try to take control of the situation as best you can. If possible, avoid places that will cause you unnecessary stress and anxiety. If you feel anxious, angry, or depressed, realize that others are experiencing similar emotions.

➤ Avoid being alone. Talk about your feelings with family or friends.

➤ Reunite with friends or family, and utilize your social and community support networks.

➤ If you have contact with children, let them know that you are there for them to talk to about the disaster and their feelings.

➤ Avoid becoming preoccupied with the disaster. Take time to get away from your "normal" routine. Find ways to distract yourself from thinking about the event and the potential for further harm. Get involved in an activity that you can control (work in the house or garden, do volunteer work, go see a movie or play).

➤ Maintain healthy behaviors. Eat a well-balanced diet. Avoid or at least minimize alcohol intake. Get regular exercise and adequate sleep. If you smoke, don't increase tobacco consumption. Although it may seem to ease anxiety in the short term, smoking has significant health risks.

➤ Learn techniques to help you relax and decrease your anxiety.

Competencies for Health Professionals in Disaster Medicine and Public Health Preparedness

Source: Subbarao I, Lyznicki J, Hsu E, et al. A consensus-based educational framework
and competency set for the discipline of disaster medicine and public health preparedness.
Disaster Med Public Health Preparedness. 2008;2:57–68.

Competency Domains	Core Competencies	Category-Specific Competencies		
		Informed Worker/Student	Practitioner	Leader
1.0 Preparation and Planning	1.1 Demonstrate proficiency in the use of an all-hazards framework for disaster planning and mitigation.	1.1.1 Describe the all-hazards framework for disaster planning and mitigation. 1.1.2 Explain key components of regional, community, institutional, and personal/family disaster plans.	1.1.3 Summarize your regional, community, office, institutional, and personal/family disaster plans. 1.1.4 Explain the purpose of disaster exercises and drills in regional, community, and institutional disaster preparation and planning. 1.1.5 Conduct hazard vulnerability assessments for your office practice, community, or institution.	1.1.6 Participate in the design, implementation, and evaluation of regional, community, and institutional disaster plans.
	1.2 Demonstrate proficiency in addressing the health-related needs, values, and perspectives of all ages and populations in regional, community, and institutional disaster plans.	1.2.1 Identify individuals (of all ages) and populations with special needs who may be more vulnerable to adverse health effects in a disaster or public health emergency.	1.2.2 Delineate health care and public health issues that need to be addressed in regional, community, and institutional disaster plans to accommodate the needs, values, and perspectives of all ages and populations. 1.2.3 Identify psychological reactions that may be exhibited by victims of all ages, their families, and responders in a disaster or public health emergency.	1.2.4 Create, evaluate, and revise policies and procedures for meeting the health-related needs of all ages and populations in regional, community, and institutional disaster plans.

2.0 Detection and Communication			
2.1 Demonstrate proficiency in the detection of and immediate response to a disaster or public health emergency.	2.1.1 Recognize general indicators and epidemiologic clues of a disaster or public health emergency (including natural, unintentional, and terrorist events). 2.1.2 Describe immediate actions and precautions to protect yourself and others from harm in a disaster or public health emergency.	2.1.3 Characterize signs and symptoms, as well as disease and injury patterns, likely to be associated with exposure to natural disasters or to conventional and nuclear explosives and/or release of biologic, chemical, and radiologic agents. 2.1.4 Explain the purpose and role of surveillance systems that can be used to detect and monitor a disaster or public health emergency.	2.1.5 Evaluate and modify policies and procedures for the detection and immediate response to natural disasters, industrial- or transportation-related catastrophes (eg, hazardous material spill, explosion), epidemics, and acts of terrorism (eg, involving conventional and nuclear explosives and/or release of biologic, chemical, and radiologic agents).
2.2 Demonstrate proficiency in the use of information and communication systems in a disaster or public health emergency.	2.2.1 Describe emergency communication and reporting systems and procedures for contacting family members, relatives, coworkers, and local authorities in a disaster or public health emergency. 2.2.2 Describe informational resources that are available for health professionals and the public to prepare for, respond to, and recover from disasters.	2.2.3 Utilize emergency communications systems to report critical health information to appropriate authorities in a disaster or public health emergency. 2.2.4 Access timely and credible health and safety information for all ages and populations affected by natural disasters, industrial- or transportation-related catastrophes (eg, hazardous material spill, explosion), epidemics, and acts of terrorism (eg, involving conventional and nuclear explosives and/or release of biologic, chemical, and radiologic agents).	2.2.5 Evaluate and modify risk communication and emergency reporting systems to ensure that health, safety, and security warnings and actions taken are articulated clearly and appropriately in a disaster or public health emergency.

(continued)

2.3 Demonstrate proficiency in addressing cultural, ethnic, religious, linguistic, socioeconomic, and special health-related needs of all ages and populations in regional, community, and institutional emergency communication systems.

2.3.1 Describe strategies for and barriers to communicating and disseminating health information to all ages and populations affected by a disaster or public health emergency.

2.3.2 Delineate cultural, ethnic, religious, linguistic, and health-related issues that need to be addressed in regional, community, and institutional emergency communication systems for all ages and populations affected by a disaster or public health emergency.

2.3.3 Create, evaluate, and revise policies and procedures for meeting the needs of all ages and populations in regional, community, and institutional emergency communication systems.

3.0 Incident Management and Support Systems

3.1 Demonstrate proficiency in the initiation, deployment, and coordination of national, regional, state, local, and institutional incident command and emergency operations systems.

3.1.1 Describe the purpose and relevance of the National Response Plan, National Incident Management System, and Hospital Incident Command System, and Emergency Support Function-8 to regional, community, and institutional disaster response.

3.1.2 Delineate your function and describe other job functions in institutional, community, and regional disaster response systems to ensure unified command and scalable response to a disaster or public health emergency.

3.1.3 Perform your expected role in a disaster (eg, through participation in exercises and drills) within the incident or emergency management system established by the community, organization, or institution.

3.1.4 Devise, evaluate, and modify institutional, community, and regional incident command, emergency operations, and emergency response systems (eg, based on after-action reports from actual events, disaster exercises, and drills) to ensure unified command and scalable response to a disaster or public health emergency.

3.2 Demonstrate proficiency in the mobilization and coordination of disaster support services.

3.2.1 Describe global, federal, regional, state, local, institutional, organizational, and private industry disaster support services, including the rationale for the integration and coordination of these systems.

3.2.2 Demonstrate the ability to collaborate with relevant public and private sector stakeholders to ensure efficient coordination of civilian, military, and other disaster response assets.

3.2.3 Develop, evaluate, and revise policies and procedures for mobilizing and integrating global, federal, regional, state, local, institutional, organizational, and private industry disaster support services in a disaster. This includes knowledge of legal statutes and mutual aid agreements for the mobilization and deployment of civilian, military, and other response personnel and assets.

3.3 Demonstrate proficiency in the provision of health system surge capacity for the management of mass casualties in a disaster or public health emergency.

3.3.1 Describe the potential impact of mass casualties on access to and availability of clinical and public health resources in a disaster.

3.3.2 Characterize institutional, community, and regional surge capacity assets in the public and private health response sectors and the extent of their potential assistance in a disaster or public health emergency.

3.3.3 Develop and evaluate policies, plans, and strategies for predicting and providing surge capacity of institutional, community, and regional health systems for the management of mass casualties in a disaster or public health emergency.

(continued)

4.0 Safety and Security				
4.1 Demonstrate proficiency in the prevention and mitigation of health, safety, and security risks to yourself and others in a disaster.	4.1.1 Using an all-hazards framework, explain general health, safety, and security risks associated with disasters. 4.1.2 Describe infection control precautions to protect health care workers, other responders, and the public from exposure to communicable diseases, such as pandemic influenza.	4.1.3 Characterize unique health, safety, and security risks associated with natural disasters, industrial- or transportation-related catastrophes (eg, hazardous material spill, explosion), epidemics, and acts of terrorism (eg, involving conventional and nuclear explosives and/or release of biologic chemical, and radiologic agents). 4.1.4 Utilize federal and institutional guidelines and protocols to prevent the transmission of infectious agents in health care and community settings.	4.1.5 Develop, evaluate, and revise community, institutional, and regional policies and procedures to protect the health, safety, and security of all ages and populations affected by a disaster or public health emergency.
4.2 Demonstrate proficiency in the selection and use of personal protective equipment at a disaster scene or receiving facility.	4.2.1 Describe the rationale, function, and limitations of personal protective equipment that may be used in a disaster or public health emergency.	4.2.2 Demonstrate the ability to select, locate, don, and work in personal protective equipment according to the degree and type of protection required for various types of exposures.	4.2.3 Develop, evaluate, and revise policies, protocols, and procedures for the use of all levels of personal protective equipment that may be used at a disaster scene or receiving facility.
4.3 Demonstrate proficiency in victim decontamination at a disaster scene or receiving facility.	4.3.1 Explain the purpose of victim decontamination in a disaster.	4.3.2 Decontaminate victims at a disaster scene or receiving facility.	4.3.3 Develop, evaluate, and revise decontamination policies, protocols, and procedures that may be implemented at a disaster scene or receiving facility.

5.0 Clinical/ Public Health Assessment and Intervention	5.1 Demonstrate proficiency in the use of triage systems in a disaster or public health emergency.	5.1.1 Explain the role of triage as a basis for prioritizing or rationing health care services for victims and communities affected by a disaster or public health emergency.	5.1.2 Explain the strengths and limitations of various triage systems that have been developed for the management of mass casualties at a disaster scene or receiving facility. 5.1.3 Perform mass casualty triage at a disaster scene or receiving facility.	5.1.5 Develop, evaluate, and revise mass casualty and population-based triage policies, protocols, and procedures that may be implemented in a disaster or public health emergency.
	5.2 Demonstrate proficiency in the clinical assessment and management of injuries, illnesses, and mental health conditions manifested by all ages and populations in a disaster or public health emergency.	5.2.1 Describe possible medical and mental health consequences for all ages and populations affected by a disaster or public health emergency. 5.2.2 Explain basic lifesaving and support principles and procedures that can be utilized at a disaster scene.	5.2.3 Demonstrate the ability to apply and adapt clinical knowledge and skills for the assessment and management of injuries and illnesses in victims of all ages under various exposure scenarios (eg, natural disasters; industrial- or transportation-related catastrophes; epidemics; and acts of terrorism involving conventional and nuclear explosives and/or release of biologic, chemical, and radiologic agents), in accordance with professional scope of practice. 5.2.4 Identify strategies to manage fear, panic, stress, and other psychological responses that may be elicited by victims, families, and responders in a disaster or public health emergency.	5.2.5 Develop, evaluate, and revise policies, protocols, and procedures for the clinical care of all ages and populations under crisis conditions, with limited situational awareness and resources.

(continued)

5.3 Demonstrate proficiency in the management of mass fatalities in a disaster or public health emergency.

5.3.1 Describe psychological, emotional, cultural, religious, and forensic considerations for the management of mass fatalities in a disaster or public health emergency.

5.3.2 Explain the implications of and specialized support services required for the management of mass fatalities from natural disasters, epidemics, and acts of terrorism (eg, involving conventional and nuclear explosives and/or release of biologic, chemical, and radiologic agents).

5.3.3 Explain the significance of (and the need to collect and preserve) forensic evidence from living and deceased humans and animals at a disaster scene or receiving facility.

5.3.4 Develop, evaluate, and revise policies, protocols, and procedures for the management of human and animal remains at a disaster scene or receiving facility.

5.4 Demonstrate proficiency in public health interventions to protect the health of all ages, populations, and communities affected by a disaster or public health emergency.

5.4.1 Describe short- and long-term public health interventions appropriate for all ages, populations, and communities affected by a disaster or public health emergency.

5.4.2 Apply knowledge and skills for the public health management of all ages, populations, and communities affected by natural disasters, industrial- or transportation-related catastrophes, epidemics, and acts of terrorism, in accordance with professional scope of practice. This includes active and passive surveillance, movement restriction, vector control, mass immunization and prophylaxis, rapid needs assessment, environmental monitoring, safety of food and water, and sanitation.

5.4.3 Develop, evaluate, and revise public health policies, protocols, and procedures for the management of all ages, populations, and communities affected by natural disasters, industrial- or transportation-related catastrophes, epidemics, and acts of terrorism.

6.0 Contingency, Continuity, and Recovery	6.1 Demonstrate proficiency in the application of contingency interventions for all ages, populations, institutions, and communities affected by a disaster or public health emergency.	6.1.1 Describe solutions for ensuring the continuity of supplies and services to meet your medical and mental health needs, as well as those of your family, office practice, institution, and community in a disaster, under various contingency situations (eg, mass evacuation, mass sheltering, prolonged shelter-in-place).	6.1.2 Demonstrate creative and flexible decision making in various contingency situations and risk scenarios, under crisis conditions and with limited situational awareness. 6.1.3 Describe community and institutional protocols and procedures for the evacuation and transport of individuals and populations (of all ages) affected by a disaster or public health emergency.	6.1.4 Develop, evaluate, and revise contingency and continuity policies and plans for health professionals, institutions, and community health systems to maintain the highest possible standards of care under various risk scenarios.
	6.2 Demonstrate proficiency in the application of recovery solutions for all ages, populations, institutions, and communities affected by a disaster or public health emergency.	6.2.1 Describe short- and long-term medical and mental health considerations for the recovery of all ages, populations, and communities affected by a disaster or public health emergency.	6.2.2 Describe solutions for ensuring the recovery of clinical records, supplies, and services to meet your physical and mental health needs, as well as those of your family, institution, and community in a disaster or public health emergency. 6.2.3 Explain mechanisms for providing postevent feedback and lessons learned to appropriate authorities (eg, through after-action reports) to improve regional, community, and institutional disaster response systems.	6.2.4 Develop, evaluate, and revise policies, plans, and procedures for the continual evaluation of regional, community, and institutional disaster response and recovery efforts, and implement necessary actions to enhance health system preparedness, response, and recovery for future events.

(continued)

7.0 Public Health Law and Ethics	7.1 Demonstrate proficiency in the application of moral and ethical principles and policies for ensuring access to and availability of health services for all ages, populations, and communities affected by a disaster or public health emergency.	7.1.1 Describe moral and ethical issues relevant to the management of individuals (of all ages), populations, and communities affected by a disaster or public health emergency.	7.1.2 Apply moral and ethical principles and policies to address individual and community health needs in a disaster. This includes understanding of professional obligation to treat, the right to protect personal safety in a disaster, and responsibilities and rights of health professionals in a disaster or public health emergency.	7.1.3 Develop, evaluate, and revise ethical principles, policies, and codes to address individual and community health needs in all disaster phases.
	7.2 Demonstrate proficiency in the application of laws and regulations to protect the health and safety of all ages, populations, and communities affected by a disaster or public health emergency.	7.2.1 Describe legal and regulatory issues relevant to disasters and public health emergencies, including the basic legal framework for public health.	7.2.2 Apply legal principles, policies, and practices to address individual and community health needs in a disaster. This includes understanding of liability, worker protection and compensation, licensure, privacy, quarantine laws, and other legal issues to enable and encourage health professionals to participate in disaster response and maintain the highest possible standards of care under extreme conditions.	7.2.3 Develop, evaluate, and revise legal principles, policies, practices, and codes to address individual and community health needs in all disaster phases.

Information Resources

Agency for Toxic Substances and Disease Registry (ATSDR):
http://www.atsdr.cdc.gov/

Located within the Centers for Disease Control and Prevention (CDC), performs specific functions concerning the effect of hazardous substances in the environment on public health. These functions include public health assessments of waste sites, health consultations concerning specific hazardous substances, health surveillance and registries, response to emergency releases of hazardous substances, applied research in support of public health assessments, information development and dissemination, and education and training concerning hazardous substances.

American Academy of Pediatrics (AAP): http://www.aap.org

National medical society dedicated to the health, safety, and well-being of infants, children, adolescents, and young adults. Members include pediatricians, pediatric medical subspecialists, and pediatric surgical specialists.

➤ **AAP Children and Disasters Web Site:**
http://www.aap.org/disasters/index.cfm

American Association of Poison Control Centers (AAPCC):
http://www.aapcc.org/DNN/

Nationwide organization of poison control centers and interested individuals. Promotes the reduction of morbidity and mortality from poisonings through public and professional education and scientific research.

American Dental Association (ADA): http://www.ada.org

Professional association of dentists committed to the public's oral health, ethics, science, and professional advancement through initiatives in advocacy, education, research, and the development of standards.

American Hospital Association (AHA): http://www.aha.org/

National organization representing all types of hospitals, health care networks, and their patients and communities. As vital community resources, hospitals must be among the best prepared, along with police, fire, rescue, and other public safety services.

American Medical Association (AMA): http://www.ama-assn.org

National professional organization for all physicians, serving as a leader of the medical profession. Through active advocacy at all levels of the private and public sectors, the AMA works to protect the patient-physician relationship, which is at the heart of medicine.

➤ **AMA Center for Public Health Preparedness and Disaster Response:** http://www.ama-assn.org/go/disasterpreparedness

➤ **AMA National Disaster Life Support™ Program Office:** http://www.ama-assn.org/go/ndls

American Nurses Association (ANA): http://www.nursingworld.org

National professional association representing the interests of the nation's registered nurses (RNs) through constituent state and territorial associations and members. This Web site provides RNs with valuable information on how they can better care for their patients, protect themselves, and prepare their hospitals and communities to respond to emergencies.

American Public Health Association (APHA): http://www.apha.org

The oldest and largest organization of public health professionals in the world. The APHA is concerned with a broad set of issues affecting personal and environmental health, including federal and state funding for health programs, pollution control, programs and policies related to chronic and infectious diseases, a smoke-free society, and professional education in public health.

American Red Cross: http://www.redcross.org/

Relief organization that assists communities across the nation during times of disaster. The Web site provides basic information on disasters, how to prepare for them, how to donate blood or money during disasters, and much more.

American Society of Health-System Pharmacists (ASHP): http://www.ashp.org/

National professional association that represents pharmacists who practice in hospitals, health maintenance organizations, long-term care facilities, home care, and other components of health care systems.

American Trauma Society: http://www.amtrauma.org/

National organization dedicated to the formation and operation of trauma systems across the country.

American Veterinary Medical Association (AVMA): http://www.avma.org

Professional association representing more than 78,000 veterinarians, who work in private and corporate practice, government, industry, academia, and the uniformed services. The AVMA produces animal-related scientific and medical information on topics such as selecting and raising a pet, protecting the public from zoonotic diseases, and developing guidelines for the proper use of lifesaving drugs in animals.

Armed Forces Radiobiology Research Institute (AFRRI):
http://www.afrri.usuhs.mil/

Institute that conducts research in radiobiology and related matters essential to the operational and medical support of the US Department of Defense and the military services. The institute collaborates with other government facilities, academic institutions, and civilian laboratories in the United States and other countries. Its findings have broad military and civilian applications.

Association for Professionals in Infection Control and Epidemiology (APIC): http://www.apic.org

Multidisciplinary, voluntary, international organization that promotes wellness and prevents illness and infection worldwide by advancing health care epidemiology through education, collaboration, research, practice, and credentialing.

Association of Public Health Laboratories (APHL): http://www.aphl.org

National organization that works to safeguard public health by strengthening public health laboratories in the United States and across the world. Public health laboratories provide diagnostic testing, disease surveillance, applied research, and laboratory training.

Association of State and Territorial Health Officials (ASTHO):
http://www.astho.org

National nonprofit organization representing the state and territorial public health agencies of the United States, the US Territories, and the District of Columbia. ASTHO members, the chief health officials of these jurisdictions, are dedicated to formulating and influencing sound public health policy and to ensuring excellence in state-based public health practice.

Centers for Disease Control and Prevention (CDC): http://www.cdc.gov

Lead federal agency for protecting the health and safety of people at home and abroad, providing credible information to enhance health decisions and promoting health through strong partnerships. The CDC serves as the national focus for developing and applying disease prevention and control, environmental health, and health promotion and education activities designed to improve the health of the people of the United States.

➤ **CDC Emergency Preparedness and Response Web Site:**
   http://emergency.cdc.gov/

Chemical Transportation Emergency Center (CHEMTREC):
http://www.chemtrec.com/Chemtrec/

Center that maintains one of the largest databases of technical information on hazardous materials. CHEMTREC provides information and assistance to physicians and other medical specialists with treatment information for acute exposures to chemicals and other hazardous materials.

Environmental Protection Agency (EPA): http://www.epa.gov/

Federal agency that works to protect human health; to safeguard the air, water, and land; and to develop and enforce regulations that implement environmental laws enacted by Congress. The agency is responsible for researching and setting national standards for a variety of environmental programs.

Department of Health and Human Services (HHS):
http://www.hhs.gov/disasters

The federal government's principal agency for protecting the health of all US citizens and providing essential human services, especially for those who are least able to help themselves.

Department of Homeland Security (DHS): http://www.dhs.gov

Department established after the terrorist attacks against the United States on September 11, 2001, to coordinate 22 previously disparate domestic agencies into one department. Its first priority is to protect the nation against further terrorist attacks. Component agencies analyze threats and intelligence, guard US borders and airports, protect our critical infrastructure, and coordinate the response to future emergencies.

➤ **DHS Ready.gov Web Site:** http://www.ready.gov

DisasterHelp.gov: http://www.disasterhelp.gov/

Multiagency federal partnership to disseminate disaster information to five overlapping audiences: (1) local/state/tribal governments, (2) individual citizens, (3) private sector businesses, (4) nongovernmental organizations (NGOs), and (5) federal agencies. This Web site supports the federal mission to provide a comprehensive, national, risk-based emergency management program of disaster mitigation, preparedness, response, and recovery, and is oriented toward helping users find information and services across a wide range of relevant disaster management topics.

Department of Transportation (DOT): http://www.dot.gov/new/index.htm

Federal department that works to ensure a fast, safe, efficient, accessible, and convenient transportation system that meets our vital national interests and enhances the quality of life of the American people.

➤ **National Highway Traffic Safety Administration:** http://www.nhtsa.gov/

➤ **Pipeline and Hazardous Materials Safety Administration, Hazmat Safety Community:** http://www.phmsa.dot.gov/hazmat

Federal Emergency Management Agency (FEMA): http://www.fema.gov

Former independent federal agency that became part of the Department of Homeland Security in March 2003. Its mission is to reduce loss of life and property and protect our nation's critical infrastructure from all types of hazards through a comprehensive, risk-based, emergency management program of mitigation, preparedness, response, and recovery.

Food and Drug Administration (FDA): http://www.fda.gov/

Agency responsible for protecting the public health by ensuring the safety, efficacy, and security of human and veterinary drugs, biologic products, medical devices, our nation's food supply, cosmetics, and products that emit radiation. The FDA is also responsible for advancing the public health by helping to speed innovations that make medicines and foods safer and more affordable, and helping the public get the accurate, science-based information it needs to use medicines and foods to improve health.

National Association of County and City Health Officials (NACCHO): http://www.naccho.org

Association engaged in several programs that collaborate with local, state, and federal partners to strengthen and improve local health agencies' capacity to respond to bioterrorism as well as communicable disease and environmental health threats.

National Association of Emergency Medical Technicians (NAEMT): http://www.naemt.org/

National professional organization dedicated to receiving and representing the views and opinions of prehospital care personnel and to influencing the future advancement of emergency medical services as an allied health profession.

National Association of EMS Physicians (NAEMSP): http://www.naemsp.org/

Organization of physicians and other professionals partnering to provide leadership and foster excellence in out-of-hospital emergency medical services.

National Association of State EMS Officials (NASEMSO): http://www.nasemsd.org/

Lead national organization for EMS, a respected voice for national EMS policy with comprehensive concern and commitment for the development of an effective, integrated, community-based, universal, and consistent EMS system.

National Disaster Life Support Foundation, Inc: http://www.ndlsf.org

Nonprofit organization composed of four academic institutions and the AMA. It serves to extend and promote the National Disaster Life Support Program and other activities in disaster medicine and public health preparedness through a national training network.

National Institute of Allergy and Infectious Diseases (NIAID):
http://www3.niaid.nih.gov/

Part of the National Institutes of Health (NIH) that conducts and supports basic and applied research to better understand, treat, and ultimately prevent infectious, immunologic, and allergic diseases.

National Institute for Occupational Safety and Health (NIOSH):
http://www.cdc.gov/niosh/topics/emergency.html

Federal agency responsible for conducting research and making recommendations for the prevention of work-related injury and illness. NIOSH is part of the CDC.

National Mental Health Association (NMHA): http://nmha.org

The United States' oldest and largest nonprofit organization addressing all aspects of mental health and mental illness. The NMHA works to improve the mental health of all Americans, especially those millions of individuals with mental disorders, through advocacy, education, research, and service.

National Voluntary Organizations Active in Disaster (NVOAD):
http://www.nvoad.org/

National organization that coordinates planning efforts by many voluntary organizations responding to disaster. Member organizations provide more effective services and less duplication in service by getting together before disasters strike. Once disasters occur, NVOAD or an affiliated state VOAD encourages members and other voluntary agencies to convene on site. This cooperative effort is a more effective way for a wide variety of volunteers and organizations to work together in a crisis.

National Oceanic and Atmospheric Administration (NOAA):
http://www.noaa.gov/

Agency that conducts research and gathers data about the global oceans, atmosphere, space, and sun. NOAA warns of dangerous weather, guides the use and protection of ocean and coastal resources, and conducts research to improve understanding and stewardship of the environment.

➤ **National Hurricane Center (NHC):** http://www.nhc.noaa.gov/

➤ **National Weather Service (NWS):** http://www.nws.noaa.gov/

National Response Center (NRC): http://www.nrc.uscg.mil/index.html

Center that serves as the sole national point of contact for reporting all oil, chemical, radiologic, biologic, and etiologic discharges into the environment anywhere in the United States and its territories. It is a joint effort of various federal agencies. The NRC Hotline national experts and federal agencies can be accessed within a few minutes (7 days a week, 24 hours a day) to provide technical assistance during a potential incident.

Nuclear Regulatory Commission (NRC): http://www.nrc.gov

Independent agency established to regulate civilian use of byproduct, source, and special nuclear materials to ensure adequate protection of public health and safety, to promote the common defense and security, and to protect the environment.

Radiological Emergency Assistance Center/Training Site (REAC/TS): http://www.orau.gov/reacts/

Organization that provides support to the Department of Energy, World Health Organization (WHO), and International Atomic Energy Agency (IAEA) in the medical management of radiation accidents. The Center's specially trained team of physicians, nurses, health physicists, radiobiologists, and emergency coordinators is prepared around the clock to provide assistance on the local, national, or international level in response to all types of radiation emergencies.

Occupational Safety and Health Administration (OSHA): http://www.osha.gov

Agency that ensures the safety and health of US workers by setting and enforcing standards; providing training, outreach, and education; establishing partnerships; and encouraging continual improvement in workplace safety and health.

Substance Abuse and Mental Health Services Administration (SAMHSA): http://www.samhsa.gov

Federal agency that works to improve the quality and availability of substance abuse prevention, addiction treatment, and mental health services. SAMHSA provides funding through block grants to states to support substance abuse and mental health services, helps improve substance abuse prevention and treatment services through the identification and dissemination of best practices, and monitors the prevalence and incidence of substance abuse.

➤ **Center for Mental Health Services (CMHS):**
http://www.mentalhealth.samhsa.gov/cmhs/EmergencyServices/default.asp

➤ **Disaster Technical Assistance Center:**
http://www.mentalhealth.samhsa.gov/dtac/default.asp

US Army Medical Research Institute of Chemical Defense (USAMRICD): http://chemdef.apgea.army.mil/

Military institute that develops medical countermeasures to chemical warfare agents and trains medical personnel in the medical management of chemical casualties.

US Army Medical Research Institute of Infectious Diseases (USAMRIID): http://www.usamriid.army.mil/

Military institute that develops medical countermeasures to biologic warfare agents and trains medical personnel in the medical management of biologic casualties.

US Fire Administration (USFA): http://www.usfa.dhs.gov/

An entity of the DHS and FEMA that seeks to reduce injuries, deaths, and economic losses from fire-related emergencies.

US Geological Survey (USGS): http://www.usgs.gov/

Federal source located within the Department of the Interior for information on the natural sciences and complex natural resource problems. Its mission is to provide reliable information to describe and understand the Earth; minimize loss of life and property from natural disasters; manage water, biologic, energy, and mineral resources; and enhance and protect our quality of life.

World Health Organization (WHO): http://www.who.int/en/

Specialized agency within the United Nations that seeks the attainment by all peoples of the highest possible level of health.

INDEX

NOTES